Experts' Perspectives on Medical Advances

This book series presents Chinese experts' perspectives on recent developments in clinical medicine. Written by leading Chinese experts in related fields, a wide variety of emerging and hot topics in internal medicine, surgery, oncology, neurosurgery, and ophthalmonology, etc., is covered by the series. Each title in this series covers a disease or a group of diseases, focusing on the basic knowledge, development and the latest research progress of clinical practice. This series is a practical and useful resource for researchers and practitioners in related subjects, as well as for general interest readers.

Ying Mao
Editor

Progress in the Diagnosis and Treatment of Gliomas

Springer

科学技术文献出版社
SCIENTIFIC AND TECHNICAL DOCUMENTATION PRESS

Editor
Ying Mao
Department of Neurosurgery
Huashan Hospital
Fudan University
Shanghai, China

ISSN 2948-1023 ISSN 2948-1031 (electronic)
Experts' Perspectives on Medical Advances
ISBN 978-981-99-0122-7 ISBN 978-981-99-0123-4 (eBook)
https://doi.org/10.1007/978-981-99-0123-4

Jointly published with Scientific and Technical Documentation Press

The print edition is not for sale in China (Mainland). Customers from China (Mainland) please order the print book from: Scientific and Technical Documentation Press.

The original submitted manuscript has been translated into English. The translation was done using artificial intelligence. A subsequent revision was performed by the author(s) to further refine the work and to ensure that the translation is appropriate concerning content and scientific correctness. It may, however, read stylistically different from a conventional translation.

This Springer imprint is published by the registered company Springer Nature Singapore Pte Ltd.
The registered company address is: 152 Beach Road, #21-01/04 Gateway East, Singapore 189721, Singapore

Foreword

In 2014, the National Central Cancer Registry of China released a report on the 10 most deadly cancers in China in 2010, with brain tumors ranking as the ninth most lethal. According to the Shanghai Municipal Center for Disease Control and Prevention, the incidence of brain tumors was found to be 7–8/100,000, higher than the national incidence rate of 5/100,000. In terms of mortality, brain tumors were the eighth most deadly cancer in women and the ninth in men. Among brain tumors, gliomas had the highest incidence, making them a significant challenge. Despite significant progress made in modern science over the past 100 years since the discovery of gliomas, particularly malignant ones, a radical cure is still elusive. Nevertheless, researchers have made significant strides in the diagnosis and treatment of gliomas in recent years, thanks to advancements in neuroimaging, anesthesiology, surgery, radiotherapy, chemotherapy, and molecular biology. Currently, the standard treatment for gliomas is a combination of surgery, radiation therapy, and chemotherapy. Thanks to progress in diagnostic and treatment technologies, the mortality rate of glioma surgery has decreased significantly, from nearly 50% in the 1950s to 1–2% in the early twenty-first century. In the Department of Neurosurgery at Huashan Hospital, Fudan University, the mortality rate is now close to zero.

Due to the infiltrative nature of glioma growth, it is challenging to remove the tumor safely without harming adjacent neural structures, even with the use of surgical microscopes. However, advances in neuroimaging, neuronavigation (including intraoperative MRI), and intraoperative electrophysiological monitoring now allow neurosurgeons to remove the tumor while safeguarding neural structures, thus improving patients' quality of life and extending their survival. Postoperative radiotherapy and chemotherapy techniques have also evolved. Intensity-modulated local radiotherapy (IMRT) has replaced conventional whole-brain radiotherapy (WBRT) to accurately irradiate tumors while preserving normal tissues based on size, location, shape, and their relationship with critical functional structures. Combining chemotherapy (such as temozolomide) with radiotherapy and administering several courses of chemotherapy after radiotherapy are also new approaches. Selective chemotherapy can be tailored to patients with different biological targets, improving treatment efficacy, avoiding inappropriate drug use, and reducing harm.

Over the past 20 years, molecular biology has significantly impacted the research, diagnosis, and treatment of glioma. The classification of gliomas has evolved from relying solely on histomorphology to a combination of histomorphology and molecular biology. Given the heterogeneity of cells within gliomas and the overlapping morphology of different types, traditional histomorphological diagnosis is not only incomplete, but also fails to reflect the tumor's biological characteristics. For instance, some patients with low-grade glioma (LGG) may survive for a long time, while others may deteriorate rapidly, similar to patients with glioblastoma multiforme (GBM), a subtype of high-grade glioma (HGG). The detection of biomarkers, such as mutations in isocitrate dehydrogenase 1 (IDH1) or IDH2, loss of heterozygosity of chromosome 1p/19q, TERT promoter mutation or IDH mutation, TP53 mutation, and ATRX mutation in LGG, and wild-type IDH in GBM, can help identify the abnormal biological behavior of tumors.

Recent biological and clinical studies have highlighted the involvement of multiple genes and steps in the development of glioma. IDH1/IDH2 mutations are considered as an early biological event in most low-grade gliomas, while other genetic alterations occur during the development of different types of gliomas. For instance, oligodendrogliomas or oligodendroastrocytomas exhibit 1p/19q loss of heterozygosity, while astrocytomas have TP53 mutations and 17p loss. Anaplastic oligodendrogliomas, anaplastic astrocytomas, and anaplastic oligodendroastrocytomas display 9p loss and RB1 pathway abnormalities. Anaplastic oligodendrogliomas and anaplastic astrocytomas have 10q and 19q loss, respectively. Incidental LGGs, which are mostly located in non-functional areas and frontal lobes, are small and exhibit IDH mutations and 1p/19q co-deletion. Our group found that patients who underwent tumor resection for incidental LGGs had a 10-year overall survival rate of 74.3%. Therefore, we believe that incidental LGGs are early-stage gliomas that can be detected early by MRI and other examinations. They should not be left untreated, as these tumors are prone to malignant transformation if they grow or become symptomatic.

After the human genome and glioblastoma genome were discovered in 2001 and 2008, respectively, some politicians and scientists optimistically predicted that a cure for glioma would be imminent. However, in reality, there is still a long way to go. In-depth research and discovery have led people to move away from unrealistic optimism towards a more rational view. The complexity and variability of transcription from gene to mRNA, and then from mRNA to protein, make it difficult to recognize proteins from a genomic standpoint. This complexity, combined with the fact that a protein must undergo at least six common modifications to express its function, has made it challenging to achieve clinical success with gene therapy for glioma. Similarly, research focused on signaling pathways has not been successful, such as Bevacizumab, a targeted therapy that was once highly anticipated. Although Bevacizumab can inhibit the vascular endothelial growth factor receptor (VEGFR) in glioma blood vessels, it can activate the c-met gene to express the MET protein in tumor cells, leading to tumor proliferation, migration, and mesenchymal transition. Key genes and signaling pathways in gliomas have yet to be identified. Fortunately, the research paradigm has shifted towards collecting large amounts of data, both laboratory and clinical, and then searching for biological patterns, rather than testing hypotheses in the laboratory.

Immunotherapy and other treatments have not been effective in significantly improving the 5-year overall survival (OS) of patients with GBM, which remains less than 10% despite high costs. The standard treatments for glioma are unsatisfactory, and gene and targeted therapies are difficult. Immunotherapy has become popular due to three main reasons: (1) gliomas are heterogeneous, with various cell clones and signaling pathways coexisting; (2) chemotherapies, such as tyrosine kinase inhibitors, antibody-based or RNA-based therapies, are unable to eliminate all tumor cell populations; and (3) tumor cells can develop drug resistance by altering signaling pathways, rendering therapies ineffective. However, immunotherapy, specifically vaccines, can activate multiple specific immune responses, altering or enhancing the immune function against tumors, and killing tumor cells, making it a promising prospect for GBM treatment. According to incomplete data, 13 clinical phase I and II trials of DC vaccines for the treatment of GBM have been completed, and 14 phase I to III trials are currently under investigation, showing mild or minimal side effects while prolonging the progression-free survival (PFS) and OS of patients to varying degrees. Another novel treatment for GBM is tumor treating fields (TTF), also known as AC electric fields (AEF), which disrupts tumor cell mitosis selectively using electric fields. The Food and Drug Administration (FDA) approved TTF for the treatment of recurrent GBM in 2011, and recent interim reports showed that combining TTF with standard therapy was more effective than standard therapy alone, resulting in PFS and OS of 7 months, 4 months, 21 months, and 16 months, respectively, ($P < 0.05$) in the treatment of primary GBM. This physical therapy results in immunogenic cell death-inducing cells, with calreticulin and high-mobility group box1 (HMGB1) depositing on the cell membrane's surface, inducing the adoptive immune response to kill the residual tumor and cancer stem cells. TTF is now included in the National Comprehensive Cancer Network (NCCN) Guidelines for CNS Cancers published in October 2015.

To conclude, while there is promise for the future of glioma treatment, there is still a considerable way to go. It is essential to continue putting forth great efforts and continually gather experience to move forward. Professor Mao Ying recognized this and quickly organized experts from the Department of Neurosurgery at Huashan Hospital, Fudan University, who have an interest in glioma research. They collected both domestic and foreign literature and combined their own experiences to create this book. The book's authors are all young surgeons and postgraduates who are actively involved in clinical work, have an academic mindset, and are knowledgeable about the latest scientific advancements. They are adept at pioneering and forging ahead. As such, this book not only reflects the current state of glioma research in China and abroad but also highlights the achievements of glioma research at

Huashan Hospital, Fudan University. It is my hope that the publication of this book will serve as a valuable reference for neurosurgeons and contribute to the treatment of glioma. I am delighted to write this at the editor-in-chief's invitation, as we welcome the New Year.

Neurosurgical Institute of Fudan University
Shanghai, China

Department of Neurosurgery
Fudan University
Huashan Hospital
Shanghai, China

Liangfu Zhou

Preface

In 1986, when I entered Shanghai Medical University (now as Shanghai Medical College, Fudan University to pursue my medical career, I could not have imagined that I would be working with the most intricate organ in the human body—the brain. Neuroscience had always awed me, as it is the most complex and uncharted field in medical studies and exploring it would require a lifetime of dedication and facing many obstacles. Despite this, I chose to embrace the challenge and delve into the unknown world of neurosurgery, where I could physically touch this enigmatic organ. Along the way, my goal has been to treat brain lesions and save the lives of my patients, making it the purpose of my life.

As a neurosurgeon, I never expected that I would choose brain tumors as the focus of my research, especially gliomas, which have a poor prognosis compared to other brain diseases. Initially, I started my work with my mentor, Academician Zhou Liangfu, treating cerebrovascular diseases. As I gained more experience and successfully performed surgeries to save stroke patients' lives by clipping cerebral aneurysms, I began to consider taking on new challenges. I contemplated whether to shift my focus towards brain tumors, specifically gliomas, and make it my new starting point, with the ultimate goal of improving the quality of life for cancer patients.

Glioma is a classic disease in neurosurgery that requires a multifaceted approach to diagnosis and treatment, including surgical skills, functional positioning, neuroimaging, and comprehensive care. With the development of new technologies, such as multimodal imaging, intraoperative MRI, intraoperative fluorescence, and intraoperative electrophysiological techniques, the diagnosis and treatment of glioma have reached new heights. Furthermore, the latest advances in molecular biology, genomics, and bioinformatics have challenged some of our outdated perspectives. As a result, new molecular typing and targeted therapies are rapidly advancing. Experts predict that there will be significant breakthroughs in the diagnosis and treatment strategies for glioma within the next decade.

Initially, my research focused on cerebrovascular diseases, and I had limited experience with glioma. At the start, I faced considerable pressure as I discovered that performing successful glioma surgery is a challenging task. However, with the support of the Shanghai spirit of "inclusiveness and pursuit of excellence" and Fudan University's school motto of "knowledge and determination, inquiring and thinking," and under the guidance and encouragement of Academician Zhou Liangfu, I began to study and explore glioma. Over the years, the concepts of glioma diagnosis and treatment have undergone constant updates and changes. Some of the previous "golden rules," such as the extent of glioma resection, the so-called silent zones surrounding the tumor, and treatment strategies after tumor recurrence, have been challenged and refreshed. This created opportunities for innovation and growth. My experience and skills in the diagnosis and treatment of cerebrovascular diseases have given me an advantage in the comprehensive care of glioma patients. Today, my experience and skills in treating both brain tumors and cerebrovascular diseases provide me with confidence and a competitive edge in my work.

Glioma's unique growth pattern and highly heterogeneous genetic background have made it a popular intersection for basic and clinical research. This book draws on the latest developments in glioma research both domestically and abroad, beginning with epidemiological research, followed by molecular pathology, genomics, and the application of new neurosurgical technologies (intraoperative MRI, navigation, etc.), as well as a comprehensive analysis of brain function. The book also covers the latest achievements in basic research and clinical treatment of glioma from the perspective of protection, advocates for the construction of MDT for glioma, and emphasizes interdisciplinary integration. This book provides a comprehensive understanding of glioma from multiple perspectives, with typical cases, rich images, texts, and novel arguments. It not only presents the author's extensive clinical work and basic research accumulation but also reflects the latest research results in the field at home and abroad. It is expected that this book will offer an academic feast for glioma researchers, and be a source of inspiration for readers, standing on their desk as a timeless reference.

This book aims to provide clinicians and basic research workers with a reference to better understand and grasp the important directions in the field of glioma research. It is hoped that the book will be beneficial to readers. Many young doctors from our department participated in writing this book, and I express my gratitude to them for their hard work. With the inspiration of the concepts of translational medicine and precision medicine, I hope that young physicians will bravely push the boundaries of research, make persistent efforts, and inherit the spirit of steadfastness, diligence, and innovation of the older generation. It is my hope that they will contribute to the advancement of glioma research.

I would like to express my gratitude to my mentor, Academician Zhou Liangfu, for his unwavering support and tolerance towards me. I am also thankful for the remarkable glioma research team that I have. They are a group of young and enthusiastic individuals who are dedicated to acquiring knowledge and are willing to complete heavy clinical work, even if it means staying late at night. Their clinical insights and understanding often provide the most pragmatic approach to glioma research, which I hope readers can appreciate in this book. As the field of glioma research is continuously evolving, and the author's proficiency is limited by time constraints, it is inevitable that some information may be omitted or out of date. Therefore, I welcome readers to provide constructive criticism and corrections.

Shanghai, China Ying Mao

Contents

Abbreviations

^{11}C-MET	^{11}C-Methionine
^{18}F-FDG	^{18}F-fluorodeoxyglucose
2-HG	2-hydroxyglutaric acid
ADCC	Antibody-dependent cell-mediated cytotoxicity
AEF	AC electric fields
AFP	Alpha-fetoprotein
AI	Artificial intelligence
ALL	Acute lymphoblastic leukemia
ALT	Alternative lengthening of telomeres
AML	Acute myeloid leukemia
APC	Antigen-presenting cell
ASL	Arterial spin labeling
BBB	Blood–brain barrier
BCG	Bacillus Calmette-Guérin
bFGF	Basic fibroblast growth factor
BMPs	Bone morphogenetic proteins
BOLD	Blood oxygenation level-dependent
CAR-T	Chimeric antigen receptor T cells
CBTRUS	Central Brain Tumor Registry of the United States
CDC	Complement-dependent cytotoxicity
CEA	Carcinoembryonic antigen
CERN	Collaborative Ependymoma Research Network
Cho/NAA	Choline/N-acetylaspartate
Chs	Cutaneous hemangiomas
CIKs	Cytokine-induced killer cells
CMV	Cytomegalovirus
CNS	Central nervous system
CSF	Cerebrospinal fluid
CSF-1	Colony- stimulating factor-1
CTA	Cancer-testis antigen
CTCs	Circulating tumor cells
CTLs	Cytotoxic T lymphocytes
DC	Dendritic cell
DCE	Dynamic contrast-enhanced perfusion imaging
DCS	Direct cortical stimulation
DIPGs	Diffuse intrinsic pontine gliomas
DSC	Dynamic susceptibility contrast

DTI	Diffusion tensor imaging
DWI	Diffusion-weighted imaging
EAP	Expanded Access Program
ECM	Extracellular matrix
ECoG	Electrode cortical graph
EEG	Electroencephalography
EGFR	Epithelial growth factor receptor
EMT	Epithelial-mesenchymal transition
ERP	Event-related potential
EVs	Extracellular vesicles
FAP	Fibroblast activation protein
FasL	Fas ligand
FDA	Food and Drug Administration
FLAIR	Fluid attenuation inversion recovery
fNIRS	Functional near-infrared spectroscopy
FRT	Fractionated radiotherapy
GBM	Glioblastoma multiforme
G-CIMP	CpG island methylator phenotype
GCP	Good Clinical Practice
G-CSF	Granulocyte-colony stimulating factor
GCV	Ganciclovir
GICs	Glioma- initiating cells
GLASS	Glioma Longitudinal AnalySiS
G-MDSC	Granulocyte-derived MDSCs
GSCs	Glioma stem cells
GWAS	Genome-wide association studies
H3-K27	Histone H3 lysine 27
HCG	Human chorionic gonadotropin
HGF	Hepatocyte growth factor
HGG	High-grade glioma
HIF	Hypoxia-inducible factor
HMGB1	High-mobility group box1
HMT	Histone methyl transferase
HPLC	High-performance liquid chromatography
HR	Hazard ratio
HRQoL	Health-related quality of life
HRV2	Human rhinovirus 2
HSV-1	Herpes simplex virus-1
IARC	International Agency for Research on Cancer
IDH	Isocitrate dehydrogenase
IDO	Indoleamine 2,3 dioxygenase
IFN	Interferon
IL-2	Interleukin-2
IMRT	Intensity-modulated local radiotherapy
IRES	Internal ribosome entry site
KLH	Keyhole limpet hemocyanin
KPS	Karnofsky Performance Scale
LAKs	Lymphokine-activated killer cells

LGG	Low-grade glioma
LITT	Laser interstitial thermal therapy
LLUMC	Loma Linda University Medical Center
lncRNA	Long-noncoding RNA
LSD1	Lysine demethylase 1
McAbs	Monoclonal antibodies
MDR	Multi-drug resistance proteins
MDSCs	Myeloid-derived suppressor cells
MDT	Multidisciplinary team
MEG	Magnetoencephalography
MEP	Motor evoked potential
METex14	MET 14exon skipping
MHC	Major histocompatibility antigen
M-MDSC	Monocyte-derived MDSCs
MMPs	Matrix metalloproteinases
MPE	Myxopapillary ependymoma
MRS	Magnetic resonance spectroscopy
MS/MS	Mass spectrometry
MV	Measles virus
NCCN	National Comprehensive Cancer Network
NO	Nitric oxide
NRP1	Neuropilin-1
NSC	Neural stem cell
NSCLC	Non-small cell lung cancer
ORR	Objective remission rates
OS	Overall survival
OV	Oncolytic viruses
PCR	Prophylactic cranial radiotherapy
PDGF	Platelet-derived growth factor
PD-L1	Programmed death ligand-1
PDT	Photodynamic therapy
PET-CT	Positron emission computed tomography
PFS	Progression-free survival
PRC	Polycomb repressive complex
PRKDC	Protein kinase catalytic subunit peptide
PRMT5	Protein arginine methyltransferase 5
PTP1B	Protein tyrosine phosphatase 1B
PV	Poliovirus
PVN	Perivascular niche
PWI	Perfusion imaging
PXA	Pleomorphic xanthoastrocytoma
rCBV	Relative cerebral blood volume
RCTs	Randomized controlled trials
ROS	Reactive oxygen species
RTK	Receptor tyrosine kinase
SDF-1	Stromal cell- derived factor-1
SDT	Soundynamic therapy
SEP	Somatosensory evoked potential

SIR	Standardized Incidence Ratio
SNPs	Single nucleotide polymorphisms
ST-EPNs	Supratentorial ependymoma
TAAs	Tumor-associated antigens
TAMs	Tumor-associated macrophages
TCGA	The Cancer Genome Atlas
TF	Tissue factor
TFP	Tissue factor pathway
TGF-β	Transforming growth factor-beta
TILs	Tumor-infiltrating lymphocytes
TK	Thymidine kinase
TMZ	Temozolomide
Treg	Regulatory T cells
TSAs	Tumor-specific antigens
TTF/TTFields	Tumor treating fields
uPA	Urokinase-type plasminogen activator
VEGFR	Vascular endothelial growth factor receptor
VM	Vasculogenic mimicry
WBRT	Whole-brain radiotherapy
WHO	World Health Organization
WIF1	Wnt inhibitory factor 1

Epidemiology and Etiology of Glioma

1

Xin Zhang, Pengji Hong, and Dongxiao Zhuang

1.1 Surge of the Incidence of Glioma

Tumors affecting the central nervous system pose a significant threat to human health. Based on data from the Central Brain Tumor Registry of the United States (CBTRUS) statistical report spanning from 2013 to 2017, the annual incidence of brain tumors is 23.79 per 100,000 individuals, with malignant brain tumors making up 7.08 per 100,000 cases and accounting for 29.80% of all brain tumors. Glioblastoma, the most common malignant brain tumor, comprises 14.50% of all brain tumors and 48.60% of malignant brain tumors. The average annual incidence of brain tumors is slightly higher in females (26.31/100,000) compared to males (21.09/100,000). Among children under 15 years of age, brain tumors have the highest incidence and mortality rates among all types of tumors. Globally, more than 256,000 people were diagnosed with malignant brain tumors in 2012, accounting for 1.80% of all malignant tumor cases. However, in China, the incidence rate is slightly higher than the global average, comprising 25.61% of all cases worldwide. As industrialization, urbanization, and aging populations continue to increase, the disease burden of benign and malignant brain and central nervous system tumors in China is rising. In 2019, China Cancer reported an estimated 101,200 new cases of brain tumors, with 47,900 occurring in males and 53,300 in females. This accounts for 2.66% of all malignant neoplasms, ranking ninth among all types of cancer (Table 1.1). The incidence of brain tumors is 7.40 per 100,000, with an accumulated incidence rate of 0.58% from ages 0 to 74. The incidence rate is higher in females than in males and in urban areas compared to rural areas. The estimated number of brain tumor-related deaths is 56,300, including 31,300 men and 25,000 women, accounting for 2.45% of all malignant tumor deaths and ranking eighth among all types of cancer. The mortality rate of brain tumors is 4.11 per 100,000, and the accumulated mortality rate from ages 0 to 74 is 0.31%. In terms of mortality rate, men have higher rates compared to women, and rural areas have higher rates than urban areas. The incidence rate of primary central nervous system tumors in Shanghai continued to increase from 1973 to 2007, rising from 3.5/100,000 and 3.03/100,000 to 5.88/100,000 and 7/100,000 in both men and women, respectively.

Neuroepithelial tumors are the most prevalent type of primary malignant tumors in the central nervous system. According to data from the United States spanning from 2011 to 2015, the annual incidence of neuroepithelial tumors is 6.57 per 100,000, representing approximately

X. Zhang · P. Hong · D. Zhuang (✉)
Department of Neurosurgery, Huashan Hospital, Fudan University, Shanghai, China
e-mail: zhuangdx@fudan.edu.cn

Y. Mao (ed.), *Progress in the Diagnosis and Treatment of Gliomas*, Experts' Perspectives on Medical Advances, https://doi.org/10.1007/978-981-99-0123-4_1

Table 1.1 Incidence rates of brain and nervous system tumors in China, 2014

Region	Sex	New cases (*10,000)	Incidence ($1/10^5$)	Composition (%)	China standard ($1/10^5$)	World standard ($1/10^5$)	Cumulative prevalence	TASR 35–64 year ($1/10^5$)
All	Population	10.12	7.40	2.66	5.63	5.55	0.58	9.16
	Male	4.97	6.83	2.27	5.40	5.32	0.54	8.40
	Female	5.33	7.99	3.15	5.86	5.76	0.61	9.95
Cities	Population	5.79	7.73	2.56	5.64	5.55	0.58	9.07
	Male	2.67	7.03	2.17	5.33	5.23	0.53	8.20
	Female	3.13	8.45	3.02	5.94	5.85	0.62	9.95
Rural	Population	4.33	7.00	2.81	5.63	5.54	0.58	9.28
	Male	2.12	6.61	2.40	5.49	5.44	0.56	8.66
	Female	2.21	7.41	3.37	5.76	5.65	0.60	9.93

TASR is the age-segmented standardized incidence rate (using the age composition of the world standard population). Data source: National Tumor Registry

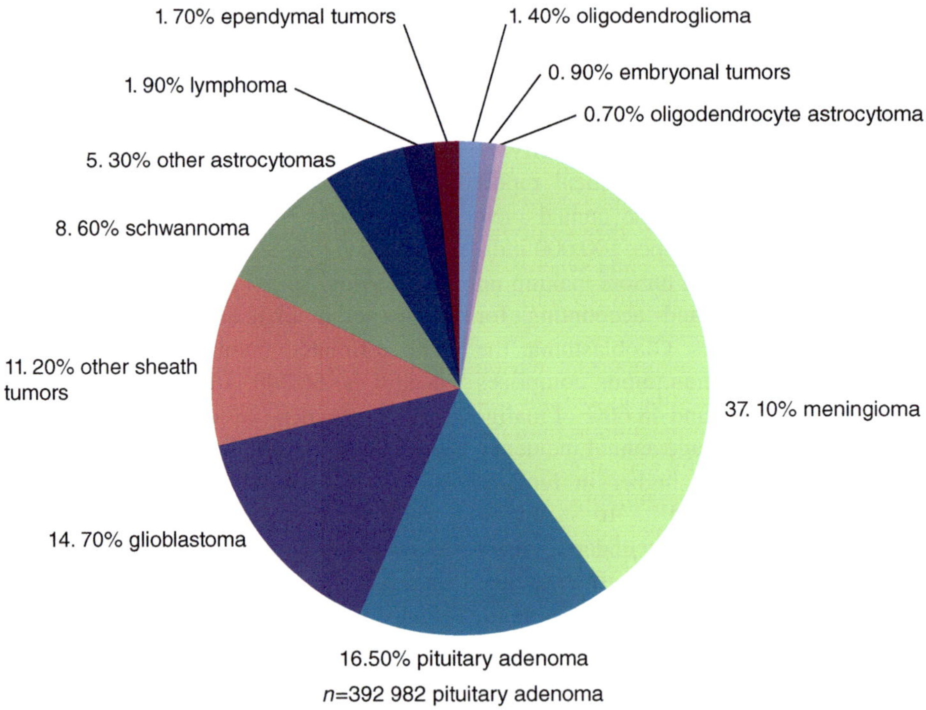

Fig. 1.1 Distribution of neurological tumors (see P003 in the main text). (Total number of cases 392,982, data source: CBTRUS 2011–2015)

28.20% of all primary brain tumors. Among these, glioblastoma has the largest proportion, accounting for 14.70% of all primary brain tumors and 47.70% of all malignant brain tumors (Fig. 1.1). In Shanghai, brain tumors accounted for 2.66% of all tumors in 2014, with an incidence rate of 12.70 per 100,000, ranking ninth among all tumors. Tumors of neuroepithelial origin accounted for 25% of primary CNS tumors in Shanghai and were more prevalent in men. From 1951 to 2011, the neuropathological department of Huashan Hospital, Fudan University, collected 38,894 primary CNS tumor specimens, of which tumors of neuroepithelial origin, meningiomas, and cranial/spinal nerve tumors accounted for 41.13%, 35.33%, and 14.43%, respectively.

Table 1.2 Genetic changes related to glioblastoma

Type of change	Incidence rate (%)	Type of change	Incidence rate (%)	Type of change	Incidence rate (%)
DNA amplification		Point mutation		Changes in gene expression	
EGFR	37	TERT	83	VEGF	Overexpression
CDE4/6	14	p53	40	Survivin	Overexpression
MDM2	11	NF1	15	SPARC	Overexpression
MDM4	7	IDH1	11	Osteopontin	Overexpression
MET	4	PIK3CA	10	CD44	Overexpression
Homozygous deletion		PIK3R1	8	IGFBP2	Overexpression
CDKN2A/B/C	47–50	MLH1、MSH2、MSH6	5	ITGAV	Overexpression
PTEN	30			HGF	Overexpression
RB1	12			PDGFA/B	Overexpression
				TGF-α	Overexpression

1.2 Glioma Is Associated with Genetics

Although the precise cause of glioma is not yet fully understood, it is widely accepted that genetic variations within a single cell are the underlying factors contributing to the development of various tumors, including glioma. Changes in specific driver genes such as point mutations, deletions, or amplifications alter the products of protein breakdown required for normal cell functioning. This, in turn, affects essential signaling pathways such as cell cycle regulation, cell proliferation, and apoptosis, leading to abnormal cell growth and eventually the formation of brain tumors. The tumor suppressor gene TP53 is often found to be mutated in both low-grade glioma (LGG) and glioblastoma (GBM). Recent studies have demonstrated that TP53/NF1 mutations implanted into Mut3 mice can induce LGG or HGG, with further induction leading to heterozygous deletion of PTEN, which accelerates the development of GBM. These findings indicate that glioma may be caused by genetic abnormalities in a single gene or multiple genes. IDH1 mutation is considered an early event in glioma development, as glioma cells with IDH1 mutation can accumulate 2-hydroxyglutaric acid (2-HG) metabolites, which are toxic to cells and can induce glioma. Glioma can also be associated with abnormalities in various genes, including EGFR, PDGFRA, CDK4/6, PTEN, NF1, TP53, CD44, TGF, VEGF, HGF, MDM2/MDM4, CDKN2A/CNKN2B, and AKT3, as shown in Table 1.2. Genomic analysis of glioma has revealed that glioma may primarily be associated with signaling pathways of receptor tyrosine kinase, Rb, and TP53. Mutated genes associated with the RB1 tumor suppressor signaling pathway were found in 77% of glioblastoma samples. Recent studies suggest that epigenetics may also play a crucial role in the development and progression of glioma. The glioma CpG island methylator phenotype (G-CIMP+) is often associated with IDH1 mutations, and patients with G-CIMP+ generally have a better prognosis than those with glioma CpG island non-methylator phenotype (G-CIMP−). Histone mutations or abnormal modifications in children with gliomas may be associated with their development, and several non-coding RNAs may also play a role in promoting or inhibiting gliomas.

1.3 X-ray May Induce Brain Tumors Including Glioma

X-rays have been identified as the sole confirmed environmental risk factor for brain tumors, including glioma. Many environments with ionizing radiation, such as occupational exposure, nuclear radiation, and radiotherapy, have been shown to cause mutations that can lead to tumors. Radiation is widely considered the most common cause of intracranial tumors, including meningiomas and sarcomas. Survivors of the atomic bombing of Hiroshima have been found to have high levels of radiation in their brains, which has been linked to an increased incidence of meningiomas, gliomas, and pituitary tumors. However, several studies have shown that children with acute lymphoblastic leukemia (ALL) have an increased risk of developing glioma after receiving prophylactic cranial radiotherapy (PCR). For example, one study analyzed 52 children with ALL who received PCR and found that six of them developed brain tumors after treatment, whereas none of the other 101 children who did not receive such treatment developed a brain tumor. A study conducted in the United States analyzed 1612 children newly diagnosed with ALL between 1967 and 1989 and found that the cumulative incidence of brain tumors during that period was 1.39%, much higher than in the general population. The study also identified 10 cases of high-grade gliomas and one case of low-grade glioma. Radiotherapy for infants and children with tinea capitis and cutaneous hemangiomas (Chs) has been found to increase the risks for schwannomas, meningiomas, and gliomas by 18%, 10%, and 3%, respectively. It has also been established clinically that secondary brain tumors are more likely to occur in patients with primary brain tumors who have previously been treated with radiotherapy. The Standardized Incidence Ratio (SIR) for patients with secondary brain tumors treated with surgery alone and those treated with radiation with or without concurrent surgery and chemotherapy were 2.0 and 5.1, respectively. Apart from the typical radiation exposure and early onset of radiation-induced gliomas, their clinical course and biological behavioral characteristics are similar to those of other types of gliomas. Low-dose radiotherapy (3–5 Gy) can also induce glioma in some patients, but the number of patients affected is often underestimated. With radiotherapy increasingly used in the treatment of intracranial tumors, patients with gliomas caused by this therapy may receive greater attention.

1.4 Relationship Between Mobile Phone Usage and Risk of Glioma

The potential relationship between mobile phone usage and the risk of glioma, has been a controversial topic for many years. While the incidence of malignant brain tumors in the United States decreased overall between 1992 and 2007, there was an increase in cases among children during this time period, which coincided with an increase in mobile phone usage among young people. Similarly, in China, the incidence of brain tumors in the Shanghai area has been increasing over the past 30 years as more people use mobile phones.

Several international institutions have conducted epidemiological studies to investigate the relationship between mobile phone usage and the risk of glioma, with the most comprehensive studies being conducted by the Hardell group and the International Agency for Research on Cancer (IARC) through their INTERPHONE study. The IARC declared radiofrequency electromagnetic field a probable carcinogen (Group 2B) to humans in 2011 based on the results of their study, which found that the risk of glioma increases in people who spend large parts of the day using mobile phones (30 min/day for 10 years). However, this result is not found in other studies, and the incidence of brain tumors has remained stable against the background of increasing mobile phone users worldwide. A case-control study conducted by the Hardell group in 2004 suggested a positive relationship between the risk of brain tumors and mobile phone usage, particularly among those aged 20–29. However, most of the odd ratios reported in this study were not statistically significant, which may have been due to the small sample size. Despite the lack of consistent evidence linking mobile phone usage and glioma risk, it is important to continue monitoring long-term data to determine whether there is a connection. A meta-analysis conducted by Gong Xiu et al. of Huashan Hospital, Fudan University, in 2014 found a positive correlation between long-term mobile phone usage on the same side of the body and the risk of glioma, particularly low-grade glioma, but no significant correlation was identified overall.

1.5 Focus on the Relationship Between Viral Infections and the Development of Glioma

Although the exact mechanism is unclear, many reports suggest that viral infections, including human cytomegalovirus (CMV), papillary polyomaviruses (such as SV40, JCV, and BKV), adenovirus, retrovirus, herpesvirus, and influenza, may have a possible association with gliomagenesis, although the role of viral infections in brain tumorigenesis has not yet been established.

Human cytomegalovirus (CMV) is a member of the herpesvirus family and is known to infect only humans, with more than 70% of adults thought to have been infected at some point in their lives. While the natural history of CMV infection involving the central nervous system in immunocompetent adults remains unclear, several studies have found CMV genomic and protein products in both tumor and blood specimens in glioma patients. One study by Mitchell et al. even found CMV genomes and proteins detectable in more than 90% of GBM tissues and 80% in peripheral blood specimens while negative in normal controls, suggesting a possible link between CMV infection and gliomagenesis. Clinical pathological studies have also shown that CMV infections in the CNS mainly affect cells in the ventricular and subventricular zones, which have a higher concentration of neural stem cells among adults. Some studies have suggested that neural stem cells are susceptible to CMV infection and that CMV infections may induce the malignant transformation of neural stem cells, leading to the dysfunction of key cellular regulatory pathways. This could result in abnormal differentiation and development of neural stem cells in the ventricular and subventricular zones, ultimately leading to the transformation of neural stem cells to glioma stem cells.

Although there is no direct evidence of CMV infections causing gliomagenesis, it is possible that in immunosuppressed patients, CMVs lurking in the microenvironment can be detected in tumor cells, neural stem cells, or glioma-associated myeloid cells. Reactivation of CMV may occur in whole or in part, and the products expressed by the reactivated virus have tumor-regulatory functions that lead to more aggressive tumors and disease progression. Recent experiments using the Mut3 transgenic mouse model of spontaneous glioma formation have supported this hypothesis. In this model, which features a genotype of GFAP-Cre; NF1flox/+; TP5+/−3, mice infected with CMV early in life showed an earlier onset of disease, lower overall survival, and higher rates of progression from grade III astrocytoma to grade IV glioblastoma compared to the control group.

While CMV infection has been detected in CD45+ monocytes within mouse tumor models, its tumorigenic effect may be mediated by the modulation of the tumor microenvironment. However, there is currently no evidence of CMV transcription mRNA in clinical sequencing studies of human tumors. Thus, further research is necessary to determine the role of CMV in gliomagenesis.

1.6 Brain Tumor Stem Cells Are Associated with Glioma Development

The concept of tumor stem cells and their role in tumorigenesis was first proposed in the 1960s. Since then, studies have revealed that cancer cells have a hierarchical composition similar to that of embryos. It has been demonstrated in vivo that a small fraction of lymphoma cells has the ability to proliferate and differentiate rapidly and that only a small fraction of these proliferating progenitor cells can replenish non-regenerating tumor cells. Therefore, tumor stem cells have been considered to be the key players in the development and tumorigenesis of tumors. This concept has subsequently been applied to other malignancies, including breast cancer, pancreatic cancer, prostate cancer, colon cancer, and brain tumors.

In recent years, researchers have discovered a subgroup of cells that can self-renew and proliferate within brain tumor tissues, playing a pivotal role in the biology of brain tumorigenesis, development, invasion, and drug resistance. These cells are called brain tumor stem cells. In the early stages of gliomagenesis, glioma stem cells overproliferate and subsequently differentiate to produce components of different differentiation levels similar to their parental tumors. Meanwhile, the stem cells themselves could proliferate but are typically maintained in a quiescent state, allowing them to escape radio- and chemotoxicity. This ultimately leads to recurrence in glioma patients after combination therapy.

Ignatova et al. identified precursor cells with neurosphere-forming ability and multipotential (neurons and astrocytes) in GBM tissues. Singh et al. confirmed these results and discovered spectrum-restricted progenitor cells with bidirectional potential in CNS tumors. These cells exhibited short-term self-renewal and could differentiate into different tumor cell subsets under specific conditions. These findings suggested the existence of tumor cells with stem cell properties among gliomas that had the ability to self-renew, proliferate infinitely, and differentiate into various cellular components of glioma. These cells were called glioma stem cells (GSCs). CD133+ and CD133− cells were isolated from GBM and implanted into NON/SCID mice, and it was found that only 100 CD133+ cells were required for tumor formation, while 50,000–100,000 CD133− cells failed to induce tumorigenesis, providing further support for the existence of GSCs.

1.7 Other Factors Associated with the Development of Glioma

Gliomas may be linked to certain familial hereditary tumor syndromes, which can result from single or multiple germline mutations or chromosomal abnormalities. According to the Mendelian theory of inheritance, these familial genetic disorders or syndromes differ from somatic mutations and can be passed on from parents to offspring, leading to a clustering of the disease in families. Examples of more common familial hereditary tumor syndromes include neurofibromatosis, Turcot syndrome, and Li-Fraumeni syndrome. Autosomal dominant neurofibromatosis types I and II result from mutations in NF1/NF2 genes, which can manifest as café-au-lait spots, plexiform neurofibromas, bilateral acoustic neuromas, gliomas, or other accompanying intracranial tumors. Turcot syndrome can arise from the loss or inactivation of MSH1, MSH2, MSH6, or PMS genes, which cause DNA mismatch or reduced DNA repair and can result in colorectal tumors and gliomas. Mutations in the oncogene TP53 can cause Li-Fraumeni syndrome, in which patients may present with multiple malignancies, including gliomas, especially in children and young adults.

The relationship between occupation and glioma remains inconclusive. Some studies suggest a higher incidence of glioma among people working in agriculture, possibly related to certain infections acquired through exposure to livestock. On the other hand, other studies have suggested that gliomas are more prevalent among white-collar workers of higher socioeconomic status in developed countries. The National Cancer Institute in the United States conducted a study that found an increased risk of glioma in various occupations, including slaughterhouse and meat processing workers, computer analysts and programmers, electricians, farmers, prosecutors, physicians, and store managers. However, there is inconsistency in these findings across different countries and regions. Interestingly, child caregivers have been found to have a lower risk of glioma.

Epidemiological data suggests a potential link between hormonal levels and tumor development, as the prevalence of meningiomas is relatively higher in females and the prevalence of gliomas is relatively lower. Researchers have examined women's endogenous and exogenous hormone levels during various times in life, such as menopause, menarche, during childbirth, and the use of oral contraceptives or hormone replacement therapy. Studies have examined age- and sex-related incidence of gliomas and meningiomas for potential associations between hormonal status and tumor development. One study suggests that gender differences in glioma incidence mainly occur between menarche and menopause, while these differences decrease among the postmenopausal age group. Another study shows an increased risk of glioma and acoustic neuroma in postmenopausal women, which contradicts data from the CBTRUS, showing a higher incidence of glioma in men in each age group, with incidence rates increasing with age in both sexes and peaking after the age of 40.

Allergies and certain immune factors have been linked to a lower risk of developing gliomas, such as asthma, hay fever, eczema, and food allergies. A meta-analysis by Linos found that allergic individuals were 40% less likely to develop gliomas. This association has also been confirmed by recent prospective studies in the United States. Additionally, several studies have demonstrated that glioma patients have lower IgE concentrations compared to control groups. The mechanisms behind the protective effects of allergies are not fully understood, but it has been suggested that inflammatory cytokines such as IL-4 and IL-13 may play a role in both allergies, autoimmune diseases, and enhanced tumor immune surveillance. Schwartzbaum found that the IL-4Rα polymorphism and the IL-13 gene increase the probability of developing allergies while decreasing the incidence of gliomas. In a case-control study among glioma patients, Wiemels found that the IL-13 SNP had similar effects while negatively correlating with IgE levels. However, no association between IL-4RαSNP and gliomas was observed. Nevertheless, studies of candidate single nucleotide polymorphisms (SNPs) have often produced false positives, and genome-wide association studies (GWAS) have not found a direct link between allergies, atopic SNP, and gliomas. Therefore, these SNP studies cannot be conclusively ruled out as an incidental coincidence.

While rare, there have been reported cases of gliomas appearing at the same site after traumatic brain injury. Although the repair mechanisms of glial cells after traumatic brain injury may be a potential factor in tumorigenesis, there is insufficient epidemiological evidence to support a clear association between the two. A meta-analysis examining the relationship between smoking and glioma development found no strong evidence supporting smoking as a risk factor for glioma.

1.8 Possibility of Extracranial Metastasis in Malignant Glioma

Recurrence of glioma is mostly limited to the site of the original tumor, but there have been rare instances of distant recurrence. Extracranial metastases are extremely uncommon, with incidence rates ranging from 0.4 to 5%, much lower than the incidence of extracranial metastases in gliosarcoma. However, recent reports have described an increasing number of cases of extracranial metastases of glioma, with metastases occurring in sites such as the bone, liver, lung, and soft tissue. One study even detected circulating tumor cells in the peripheral blood of glioma patients, providing evidence for the mechanism of extracranial metastasis of glioma through the bloodstream.

The tumor microenvironment may temporarily disrupt the blood–brain barrier, allowing tumor cells to spread through the bloodstream and establish distant metastases. While only a small percentage of tumor cells evade the immune system and form extracranial metastases, recent reports suggest that this phenomenon is increasing. In addition to blood-borne metastases, there have also been cases of glioma developing in the skull and scalp near the surgical site, potentially due to iatrogenic contamination. There have even been cases of glioma developing in transplanted organs from donors with GBM. Although the likelihood of extracranial metastasis in glioma is lower compared to other malignancies, advances in treatment and prolonged survival of glioma patients may pose new challenges in diagnosis and treatment in the future.

Further Reading

Bao P, Gong YM, Peng P, et al. Analysis of malignant tumor incidence and mortality characteristics in Shanghai in 2014. China Oncol. 2018;28(3):161–76.

Brennan CW, Verhaak RG, McKenna A, et al. The somatic genomic landscape of glioblastoma. Cell. 2013;155(2):462–77.

D'Elia A, Tropeano MP, Maiola V, et al. The etiology of low-grade gliomas: pathological and clinical considerations about radiation-induced low-grade gliomas. Neurol Sci. 2015;36(7):1091–5.

Gong X, Wu JS, Mao Y, et al. A meta-analysis of the relationship between mobile phone use and glioma incidence. Chin J Med. 2014;94(39):3102–6.

Han RQ, Zhou JY, Zheng RS, et al. Analysis of brain tumor incidence and mortality in China in the year 2014. China Cancer. 2019;28(3):161–6.

Kexin S, Siwei Z, Rongshou Z, et al. Analysis of malignant tumor incidence and mortality by region in China in the year 2015. China Cancer. 2019;28(1):1–11.

Liangfu Z. Modern neurosurgery. 2nd ed. Shanghai: Fudan University Press; 2015.

Ostrom QT, Bauchet L, Davis FG, et al. The epidemiology of glioma in adults: a "state of the science" review. Neuro Oncol. 2014;16(7):896–913.

Ostrom QT, Gittlema NH, Truitt G, et al. CBTRUS statistical report: primary brain and other central nervous system tumors diagnosed in the United States in 2011–2015. Neuro Oncol. 2018;20(suppl_4):iv1–iv86.

Samkange-Zeeb F, Schlehofer B, Schüz J, et al. Occupation and risk of glioma, meningioma and acoustic neuroma: results from a German case–control study (Interphone study group, Germany). Cancer Epidemiol. 2010;34(1):55–61.

Shen F, Wu CX, Yao Y, et al. Transition over 35 years in the incidence rates of primary central nervous system tumors in Shanghai, China and histological subtyping based on a single center experience spanning 60 years. Asian Pac J Cancer Prev. 2013;14(12):7385–93.

Winn HR. Youmans neurological surgery. 7th ed. WB Saunders; 2017.

Zhou B, Liu W. Post-traumatic glioma: report of one case and review of the literature. Int J Med Sci. 2010;7(5):248–50.

2 Advances in Molecular Classification of Gliomas

Zhifeng Shi

Glioma is the most prevalent malignant tumor of the central nervous system, and current standard therapies involve surgery combined with radiotherapy and/or chemotherapy. However, the response to treatment and overall prognosis would vary among individuals, confusing for clinicians. Fortunately, the rapid development of gene sequencing technology in this century has provided a deeper understanding of the gene profile of human glioma through large-scale and high-throughput sequencing. This has enabled the implementation of precision medicine, providing a basis and direction for individualized treatment. Molecular classification has become an important part of pathological diagnosis, and an integrated diagnosis report with both molecular and histology components has been released in the most recent WHO CNS5 glioma classification scheme. Understanding molecular classification and diagnosis of glioma can aid clinicians in accurately determining the prognosis of patients and providing personalized treatment.

The discovery of four genetic events—1p/19q co-deletion, MGMT promoter methylation, IDH1/IDH2 mutation, and TERT promoter mutation—marks a significant milestone in the molecular classification of gliomas. These indicators are highlighted in the CNS5 edition and have been used as references for judging the efficacy of various studies and clinical trials at present. A worldwide multicenter collaboration has established a unified glioma biospecimen repository, along with standard biospecimen processing procedures, high-quality genetic sequencing platforms, and molecular classification systems. Several classification schemes have been developed, including the three-type classification scheme for GBM by Phillips et al. the six-type classification scheme for glioma by Li et al. the four-type classification scheme for GBM by the Cancer Genome Atlas (TCGA), the two-type classification scheme for WHO grade II and III by Zhang et al. and the three-type classification scheme for GBM by Professor Jiang Tao. Although these schemes may differ in opinion, they all have a theoretical basis and clinical guidance.

2.1 Molecular Classification of Glioblastoma

Phillips et al. have classified high-grade GBM into three types: proneuronal (enriched in neurogenesis-related markers), proliferative (enriched in cell proliferation-related markers), and mesenchymal (enriched in mesenchymal tissue and blood vessels). Prognosis differs significantly between these types, with the latter two having a relatively poor prognosis. In 2009, the TCGA, funded by NIH and initiated as a genomic

Z. Shi (✉)
Department of Neurosurgery, Huashan Hospital, Fudan University, Shanghai, China
e-mail: shizhifeng@fudan.edu.cn

Y. Mao (ed.), *Progress in the Diagnosis and Treatment of Gliomas*, Experts' Perspectives on Medical Advances, https://doi.org/10.1007/978-981-99-0123-4_2

study, included GBM as one of the first three malignancies to be studied. The study analyzed over 200 GBM cases and examined genome sequencing, methylation, mRNA expression, miRNA expression, among others. The results revealed three primary cancer signaling pathways altered in GBM, including the RTK pathway (88%), P53 pathway (87%), and Rb tumor suppressor pathway (78%). Through bioinformatics analysis, GBM has been classified into four distinct molecular subtypes: proneural, neural, classical, and mesenchymal. Each subtype has unique biological and clinical characteristics, such as IDH1 mutation and PDGFRA amplification/high expression being predominantly found in the proneural subtype, while 97% of the classical subtype exhibits EGFR amplification. Several well-known oncogenes, including TP53, PTEN, NF1, CDNK2A, and LZTR1, were also involved in these subtypes. The development of antibodies against proteins expressed by these genes, such as IDH R132H, enables simple immunohistochemical testing, which can replace costly second-generation sequencing. This development provides convenient clinical patient risk stratification and treatment screening. The proneural subtype is generally associated with younger patients and a better prognosis, while the mesenchymal subtype has the worst prognosis but is more responsive to immunotherapy. Patients with the classical subtype can benefit from intensive therapy, which involves temozolomide (TMZ) combined with more than three courses of adjuvant chemotherapy, but this treatment approach has little value for patients with the proneural subtype. Similar results were obtained by Prof. Jiang Tao and his team at Beijing Tiantan Hospital, Capital Medical University, who conducted the same study on GBM in the Chinese population and identified three subtypes (G1, G2, and G3) with biological and clinical characteristics consistent with the four subtypes identified by TCGA. This underscores the importance of molecular classification for GBM and provides a valuable platform and genetic-biological resource for in-depth study and comprehensive understanding of the disease. As more samples were enrolled in TCGA, it became evident that epigenetics plays an equally significant role in GBM, with methylation being the most prominent type.

In previous report, a specific methylation subtype was identified in GBM known as the glioma CpG island methylation phenotype (G-CIMP). Patients with this subtype tend to be younger and have a better prognosis. It is worth noting that CpG island methylation (CIMP) of these genes can be a secondary event to IDH mutation. The TCGA is continuing to update its sample pool with over 700 cases and has made several important new findings, such as the significance of gene rearrangements and telomerase, and the discovery that MGMT promoter methylation is most relevant in classical subtypes. However, different classification systems can complement each other and maintain their unique differences during mutual integration. For example, Professor Fan Xiaolong's group from Beijing Normal University's College of Life Sciences, in collaboration with Professor Jiang Tao's group from Beijing Tiantan Hospital of Capital Medical University and Lund University in Sweden, proposed a molecular co-expression network-based glioma classification system. This system clearly classifies glioma samples into three major groups based on EGFR and PDGFRA, each containing 30–40 core genes that do not overlap with each other. This finding differs slightly from previous TCGA analyses. Nevertheless, advancements in technology will inevitably lead to more glioma subtypes, and the current challenges in molecular classification of glioma will become clearer in the future.

Molecular classification has enabled the study of inter-individual genetic heterogeneity in GBM, but it also faces some challenges. For instance, Sottoriva et al. collected intraoperative tumor multi-locus specimens and conducted deep sequencing in 11 GBM patients, using the TCGA classification as a reference, and found different molecular subtypes within the same tumor. Similarly, a study conducted by MD Anderson, which performed genomic and epigenetic studies on multicenter GBM, revealed significant differences in the molecular genetic background of multicenter GBM and single-center GBM.

Kim et al. identified spatial and temporal changes in genomics during GBM recurrence, with more driver genetic changes in distantly located recurrent tumors than in locally recurrent tumors. Van den Bent et al. found that approximately half of patients with 55 primary/recurrent paired GBM showed deletion of epidermal growth receptor type III mutant (EGFRvIII) expression after recurrence. Our group studied 57 IDH mutant GBM cases in Huashan Hospital and found that they could be divided into G-CIMP high expression and G-CIMP low expression subgroups. CDKN2A deletion was the most common copy number variation and was significantly correlated with G-CIMP low expression. G-CIMP low expression, CDKN2A deletion, and MET amplification were associated with poor overall survival time. Therefore, we stratified IDH mutant glioblastoma into three molecular subgroups: Group 1 (G-CIMP high expression), Group 2 (G-CIMP low expression without CDKN2A or MET alteration), and Group 3 (G-CIMP low expression with CDKN2A and/or MET alteration). Group 1 and 2 have a relatively good prognosis, but we observed that Group 3 exhibited quite a poor overall survival time. After finding genetic heterogeneity in IDH mutant GBM, we hypothesized that IDH mutant GBM may not be confined to a secondary tumor; IDH mutant primary GBM might be an individual tumor entity. We recruited 67 IDH mutant primary GBM/astrocytoma IV cases without prior low-grade glioma in our early study. Typical molecular alterations such as TERTp mutation, EGFR amplification, and combined +7/−10 were rarely seen in this cohort. DNA methylation classification indicated that these tumors belong to the IDH mutant high-grade astrocytoma subclass. G-CIMP subgroups, MGMT promoter methylation, and TP53 mutation are useful prognostic adjuncts. Classical GBM is characterized by IDH wild type and TERTp mutation; however, approximately 20% of IDH wild-type GBM is combined with TERTp wild type, which we call triple negative GBM. Hai Yan et al. studied the genomic landscape of IDH/TERTp wild-type GBM and found two genetic subgroups characterized by TERT-structural rearrangements and ALT-positive with mutations in ATRX or SMARCAL1. However, such genetic subgrouping shows limited correlation with patients' clinical outcomes.

2.2 Molecular Classification of Lower-Grade Gliomas

The WHO 2007 classification of brain tumors defines grade I–II gliomas as LGG and grade III–IV gliomas as HGG. However, with the advancement of molecular genetics of gliomas, grade II–III gliomas are now more commonly referred to as LGG. Following a large-scale genomics study of GBM, LGG genomics studies have received more attention. This is because lower-grade gliomas may be early events in glioma development and progression, and studying these tumors can provide a clearer understanding of malignant progression. Furthermore, patients with lower-grade gliomas have a better overall prognosis and may be the first glioma type to be targeted in the future. In 2015, the TCGA, German Glioma Collaborative Group, and Japanese Glioma Collaborative Group published genomics studies on lower-grade gliomas after years of effort. The findings of all three studies were largely consistent. Unlike GBM, lower-grade gliomas have a clearer biogenetic signature and molecular classification, which may be related to their location close to the trunk and having fewer branches, according to the "big tree theory" of tumor microevolution. The importance of IDH1/2 mutation, TERT promoter (TERTp) region mutation, and 1p/19q co-deletion is emphasized in all three studies, which dominate the genotyping of lower-grade gliomas. Tumors with IDH1/2 mutation/TERT mutation/1p19q co-deletion are called "triple positive," while those without are called "triple negative." The classification of lower-grade gliomas also includes IDH1/2 mutant, IDH1/2/TERT double mutant, and TERT mutant types, resulting in a total of five categories. This classification correlates with the histopathologic classification, in which "triple positive" is predominantly seen in oligodendrogliomas, which have the best prognosis and contain mutations in the CIC and FUBP1 genes.

Conversely, "triple-negative" and TERT mutant types are frequently observed in GBM, which have the worst prognosis and feature chromosome 7 and 19 amplifications and deletions of CDNK2A/B and PTEN. The IDH1/2 mutant type is mainly found in astrocytoma, which has an average prognosis and typically presents mutations in the ATRX and TP53 genes. The survival expectation of glioma patients under conventional histopathological diagnosis can vary greatly, and even low-grade gliomas may show early recurrence and death. To more accurately determine the prognosis of low-grade glioma patients, molecular diagnosis is becoming increasingly important. New criteria and classification methods will be necessary to achieve a more accurate understanding of glioma.

2.3 Molecular Diagnosis of Glioma Based on Molecular Markers Challenges Traditional Theories

As previously mentioned, large-scale, high-throughput sequencing technology has ushered in the era of "big data" in the study of gliomas. While this has broadened our understanding of the molecular genetic background of gliomas, it has also posed challenges in identifying the key factors that determine glioma occurrence and development in this vast sea of information, hindering the translation of precision medicine into clinical practice. In the past, glioma diagnosis relied solely on histopathology, which had inherent subjective biases due to interobserver differences among pathologists. A study conducted in the United States asked different pathologists to diagnose the same group of glioma cases to assess the consistency of pathological diagnoses. Shockingly, 45% of the cases had diagnostic differences, and even after a second review, 27% of the cases still had inconsistencies, leading to erroneous prognosis and treatment planning. Therefore, many researchers have sought to identify critical molecular markers in glioma development to improve the accuracy of molecular diagnosis and achieve the clinical application of "From Bench to Bedside." One of the most notable findings in the field of glioma research comes from Prof. Yan Hai at Duke University, who discovered extensive mutations in the TERTp region gene in gliomas. Combining this discovery with mutations in the IDH1/IDH2 genes enabled direct pathological diagnosis of gliomas, which correlated well with conventional histopathological diagnosis. In Prof. Yan's study cohort, simultaneous mutations in IDH1/2 and TERT genes were common in oligodendrogliomas, while IDH1/2 mutation/TERT wild type tended to be astrocytoma, and IDH1/2 wild type/TERT mutation was considered for oligodendroglioma, with the remainder being oligoastrocytoma. While this finding holds promise for molecular diagnosis, some experts remain skeptical of relying solely on two molecular indicators for pathological diagnosis. Even for a single molecular subtype, such as IDH1 mutation in lower-grade glioma, there can be variations in patients' clinical prognosis, indicating that a single molecular marker is not sufficient for precise molecular diagnosis. Additional molecular markers will be needed in the future, and a "marker array" may be employed to reduce errors and bias in molecular diagnosis.

The 1p/19q co-deletion has been a widely recognized marker of oligodendroglioma. Patients with this deletion are responsive to chemotherapy and have a better prognosis. In a study by the Bettegowda group, CIC mutations were found on 19q in six out of seven cases of oligodendroglioma, and FUBP1 mutations were found on 1p in two out of seven cases. CIC mutations were also found in 12 out of 28 validation cases, while FUBP1 mutations were found in three cases. The discovery of these two genes is believed to be crucial for understanding the molecular biology and pathological changes of oligodendroglioma. The significance of CIC and FUBP1 mutations in oligodendroglioma with 1p/19q co-deletion was further explored by Prof. Ng Ho-keung of the Chinese University of Hong Kong. It was found that patients with oligodendroglioma with 1p/19q co-deletion had a better prognosis, but those with CIC or FUBP1 mutations had a worse prognosis than those with CIC or FUBP1 wild type. These mutations can be detected by immunohistochemistry, providing an essential basis for further molecular classification of oligodendrogliomas in the future. However, the discovery of these mutations raises a new question: whether chemotherapy combined with radiotherapy is necessary for oligodendrogliomas with 1p/19q co-deletion and CIC or FUBP1 mutations. This question needs to be verified through clinical trials. Similarly, Prof. Yan Hai's study on anaplastic astrocytoma using exon sequencing revealed the presence of IDH1 mutation (75%), ATRX mutation (63%), and TP53 mutation (82%), which are rarely found in GBM. These mutations are believed to be key factors leading to the progression of tumor cells to astrocytes.

The TCGA integrated analysis of genomic data from high-grade and lower-grade gliomas highlights the significance of key genetic events in determining the glioma spectrum. For instance, if IDH1 is wild type, primary GBM is predominantly present with PTEN, NF1, CDNK2A deletion, EGFR amplification, and TERTp mutation. On the other hand, if IDH1 mutation with 1p/19q co-deletion is present, oligodendroglioma with CIC, FUBP1, and TERTp mutations is predominant.

Oligoastrocytoma could be clearly classified as either oligodendroglioma or astrocytoma with molecular diagnostic techniques, eliminating the need for the diagnosis of oligoastrocytoma.

2.4 Age Has a Huge Impact on the Molecular Classification of Gliomas

It is evident that the prognosis of glioma patients tends to worsen with age, as seen in various studies that have focused on gliomas in both elderly and adolescent populations. Molecular classification also reveals unique features in these specific age groups. However, due to their low incidence and insufficient attention, conventional molecular classification methods, such as the GBM classification of TCGA, do not provide a separate classification for these groups.

1. Elderly glioma: The definition of elderly age varies, with three broad categories (>60 years, >65 years, and >70 years). Patients with gliomas that develop at the age of ≥60 years are commonly referred to as elderly gliomas. Unfortunately, their overall prognosis is poor, with a median survival of only 4 months in half of the patients. This is due in part to the disease itself but also to the physical condition of the patients. Elderly patients may have declining cognitive function, which can lead to misdiagnosis due to memory loss and psychiatric symptoms. While extensive surgical resection combined with postoperative radiotherapy is often recommended to improve the prognosis of GBM in the elderly, many elderly patients have severe chronic obstructive pulmonary disease, cardiovascular disease, and other disorders that make them less tolerant of the perioperative period. Therefore, it is important to carefully weigh the advantages and disadvantages of surgery, radiotherapy, and chemotherapy for elderly patients, as well as their impact on neurological functions such as cognition after surgery. Conventional chemotherapeutic drugs are not recommended as the first choice of adjuvant therapy for elderly glioma patients due to their high adverse effects. Instead, simultaneous radiotherapy with postoperative TMZ is commonly recommended both in China and aboard. If the body condition of the patient does not allow for high-dose radiotherapy, oral TMZ alone may be recommended. In this process, MGMT promoter methylation still plays an important role in predicting TMZ sensitivity in elderly glioma patients, as it does in adult glioma patients. Additionally, frailty is a common pathophysiological process in the elderly. Some studies have found that the frailty index is an independent factor affecting the prognosis of GBM in the elderly, with frail elderly GBM patients having longer hospital stays and a worse prognosis.
2. Young adult gliomas: Compared to adult and elderly gliomas, young adult gliomas have a unique genetic background with some mutations occurring only in adolescents. A

2015 report on pediatric and young adult gliomas found significant genetic differences between these two types of gliomas. Childhood gliomas are predominantly GBM, with relatively few LGG, and the genetic differences between childhood GBM and adult GBM are significant. The German Cancer Research Center conducted a retrospective analysis of 202 cases of GBM in children (1–18 years) and found that GBM in children can be divided into three subtypes based on methylation levels and molecular background: a subtype similar to lower-grade adult gliomas; a subtype similar to adult pleomorphic xanthoastrocytoma (PXA), mostly containing the BRAF V600E mutation and CDKN2A heterozygous deletion; and a subtype typical of GBM in children. The prognosis of tumors with a similar genetic background to lower-grade gliomas is the best, followed by PXA, and worst for GBM. Using K27M and oncogene amplification as risk factors, children GBM can be classified as "intermediate risk" or "high risk": "intermediate risk" includes G34R/IDH1 mutation, MGMT promoter methylation, and low-grade glioma-like, and PXA-like, with a 3-year survival rate over 70%, while the "high risk" includes K27M mutation and oncogene amplification, with a 3-year survival rate no more than 5%. This result gives us a new understanding of HGG in children and allows us to make an accurate judgment about the prognosis of GBM in children. Although LGG in children is rare, it does have very characteristic molecular alterations. A retrospective analysis of 886 children LGG cases by Professor Tabori in Canada, funded by the "Pediatric Low Grade Glioma Foundation," found a low rate of progression to HGG (2.9%), but a high rate of BRAF V600E mutation and CDNK2A deletion in patients who progressed to HGG. This genetic alteration helps to distinguish primary from secondary HGG in children and may suggest that LGG in children is more likely to progress to HGG if the BRAF V600E mutation and CDNK2A deletion are present. However, in cases that progress to HGG, the time to malignancy is longer than in the wild type if the BRAF V600E mutation is present (6.65 years vs. 1.59 years), with a higher 5-year survival rate. Young adult GBMs also have different genetic backgrounds. The author conducted a retrospective analysis of 108 cases of GBM in young adults (18–35 years) and found a high proportion of BRAF V600E, H3F3A, and IDH1 mutations, which were 15%, 15.9%, and 16.8%, respectively. The study directly classified young adult GBM into BRAF mutant types, H3F3A mutant types, and IDH1 mutant types, among which BRAF mutant type patients were younger, had easier surgical resection and better prognosis, and usually had CDNK2A deletion. However, in the TCGA database, the BRAF mutation rate in adult GBM and elderly GBM is extremely low (<2%), which suggests that gliomas of different ages may have different cellular origins, resulting in distinct genetic backgrounds.

Besides, pediatric gliomas have been redefined in WHO CNS5, which are separated from adult gliomas now.

2.5 Molecular Diagnosis and Treatment of Glioma

Thanks to the numerous molecular biology studies, the molecular genetic background of glioma is now better understood, and the WHO glioma diagnostic criteria is being revised to include molecular diagnosis. At the Haarlem meeting before the 2016 WHO annual meeting, there was a consensus that molecular diagnosis would alter the traditional pathological diagnosis of glioma from "astrocytoma, oligodendroglioma, oligoastrocytoma, and GBM" to "GBM, IDH mutant GBM, IDH mutant astrocytoma, IDH wild-type astrocytoma, and oligodendroglioma." Immunohistochemistry can detect IDH1, ATRX, and TP53 mutations, making molecular diagnosis more applicable in clinical settings. For example, IDH1 immunohistochemistry staining is performed firstly, and those who are negative are classified as IDH wild-type astrocytoma and GBM; those who are IDH1 positive then undergo ATRX immunohistochemistry staining, and if ATRX expression is absent, then the diagnosis is considered to be a classical astrocytoma. If ATRX expression is positive, then 1p/19q deletion testing is performed, and if there is co-deletion, the diagnosis is considered to be oligodendroglioma and IDH mutant GBM if intact. Kim et al. discovered that the genomics of GBM recurrences were less likely to develop hypermutations in IDH1 wild-type primary GBM after standardized treatment, which provides guidance for the clinical treatment of IDH1 wild-type GBM with local recurrence in situ and may also impact glioma prognosis and the development of personalized radiotherapy regimens, laying the groundwork for precise glioma treatment.

The role of molecular diagnosis in routine glioma diagnosis was firstly indicated by WHO (2016), and it has now become an official component of the final pathological report according to the updated WHO (2021) CNS5. The report will consist of four layers: integrated diagnosis, histological diagnosis, WHO grade, and molecular information, such as IDH1 mutant, 1p19q co-deletion, oligodendroglioma, WHO 2. Molecular classification has proven to be a more reliable predictor of the prognosis of glioma patients than histological diagnosis. Huashan neurosurgical team collaborated with Prof H K Ng CUHK to develop a single-gene-based molecular stratification scheme, using IDH1/2, 1p19q, H3, BRAF, EGFR, 10q examined in a cohort of 1028 adult gliomas. Totally, 6 molecular subgroups are generated with Group 1 (1p19q co-deletion, IDH mutation), Group 2 (IDH mutation, 1p19q non-co-deletion, TERTp mutation), Group 3 (IDH mutation, 1p19q non-co-deletion, TERTp wild type), Group 4 (IDH wild type, BRAF mutation), Group 5 (IDH wild type, BRAF wild type, and not possessing the criteria of Group 6), and Group 6 (IDH wild type, any one of TERTp mutation, EGFR amplification, H3 mutation, or 10q deletion). Group 1 patients have the best overall survival time, while Group 6 patients exhibit the worst overall survival time. Such a molecular classification system is more feasible to routine clinical practice.

Molecular diagnosis can provide insight into the course of glioma malignant transformation. In the GLASS (Glioma Longitudinal AnalySiS) study, Souza et al. performed DNA methylation sequencing on IDH1/2 mutant gliomas and found that changes in G-CIMP expression pattern after treatment, from high to low expression, indicate that patients may benefit less from adjuvant treatment and have shorter survival after tumor recurrence. Additionally, Capper et al. developed a novel diagnostic technology in 2018 using methylation sequencing for some hard-to-diagnose cases. However, due to its high cost and complex analysis technology, it is not recommended for routine diagnosis procedures.

Gene fusion is an important component of gene mutation that plays a crucial role in the molecular diagnosis and treatment of glioma. In 2009, Singh et al. reported the presence of the FGFR-TACC fusion gene in gliomas, and subsequent studies have shown that GBM with this fusion gene is highly aggressive. In Paris, France, Professor Anna Luisa Di Stefano of Sorbonne University General Hospital used this fusion gene as a target for JNJ-42756493-targeted therapy in two patients with recurrent GBM and positive FGFR3-TACC3 fusion gene. The patients showed significant tumor shrinkage on imaging, indicating that FGFR-TACC may establish a new subtype of GBM and become a potential therapeutic target. In China, Su Xiaodong and Jiang Tao et al. sequenced 272 cases of WHO grade II, III, and IV and recurrent glioma samples, verified the above fusion genes, and reported a new fusion gene PTPRZ1-MET (ZM) in cMET for the first time. ZM has the following characteristics: (1) it can be mutually exclusive with EGFR amplification events and is not associated with IDH1 mutation; (2) MET, PIK3CA, AKT1, and other genes in ZM samples are highly expressed, suggesting activation of the PIK3CA pathway; (3) ZM enables higher cell migration and invasive capacity of glioma cells; (4) among patients with recurrent GBM, those with ZM have a worse prognosis. These findings provide a theoretical basis for molecularly targeted therapies. EGFR amplification and overexpression, as well as its mutation (EGFRv III), frequently occur in GBM, and both can act as receptor tyrosine kinase (RTK) to induce downstream signaling pathways (e.g., Ras, PI3K, etc.); promote tumor proliferation, invasion, and metastasis; and induce resistance to radiotherapy/chemotherapy. Although antitumor drugs targeting tyrosine receptors have entered clinical phase I, II, and III, the clinical results in glioma have not been as good as expected.

A phase I/II study of gefitinib by Chakravarti et al. did not demonstrate any benefit over radiotherapy alone, and clinical trials of erlotinib in combination with TMZ chemotherapy and radiotherapy for primary GBM showed high adverse effects without significant efficacy. Dose-limiting adverse effects such as rash, pulmonary embolism, and neutropenia have also been reported in studies using erlotinib alone. Despite these unsatisfactory results, ongoing phase I and II clinical trials are still exploring the use of EGFR inhibitors, such as BIBW2992, in combination with TMZ and/or radiotherapy for the treatment of malignant gliomas. Further adaptation and optimization are needed to improve the efficacy and safety of these treatments.

The initial data of The Cancer Genome Atlas (TCGA) in 2008 were obtained from Affymetrix Human Exon 1.0 ST Gene Chips, Affymetrix HT-HG-U133A Gene Chips, and custom-designed Agilent 244,000-feature gene expression microarrays. Over the past 6 years, rapid technological advances have led to constant upgrades in sequencing methods and the discovery of new candidate genes with varying levels of expression, existence states, and spatial and temporal distributions. The molecular classification of gliomas has also evolved toward a more precise "pyramidal" approach. The genetics-based molecular pathological classification has compensated for the previous poor judgment of prognosis and clinical features, providing stronger clinical guidance. Our understanding of the heterogeneity of glioma biological behavior has changed from "foggy" to "clear." However, the critical question remains: how can we use these results to provide more precise treatment to patients? While accurate diagnosis of glioma has advanced rapidly, precision treatment after diagnosis remains insufficient. It is crucial for neurosurgeons, particularly neuro-oncologists, to better connect diagnosis and treatment.

2.6 Molecular Classification of Medulloblastoma Is the Way Forward

Medulloblastoma, which was named as early as 1925, is one of the most common malignancies in children. Pathologically, there are five major types of medulloblastoma: classic medulloblastoma, large cell medulloblastoma, anaplastic medulloblastoma, desmoplastic medulloblastoma, and extensive nodular medulloblastoma. The prognosis of medulloblastoma is judged by risk factors such as tissue type, age, and whether the tumor spreads, which guide the development of subsequent radiotherapy regimens. With the development of chemotherapeutic agents and radiotherapy, the clinical cure rate of medulloblastoma has been increasing, and the clinical prognosis has significantly improved. Although medulloblastoma is not a glioma, as a malignant brain tumor, it shares many similarities with glioma. In recent years, the "Medulloblastoma Research Collaborative Network," led by Michael Taylor in Canada, has initiated large sample, high-throughput gene sequencing of medulloblastoma and transcriptional expression profiling. Medulloblastoma is divided into four subtypes at the molecular level: WNT, SHH, Group 3, and Group 4. Each of the molecular subtypes of medulloblastoma has distinct genetic, demographic, and clinical features, which offer a precise foundation for more accurate risk stratification and molecularly targeted therapy in the future.

WNT medulloblastoma is characterized by alterations in the WNT/β-catenin signaling pathway and is the least common of the four molecular subtypes. Typical molecular alterations include chromosome 6 deletion, CTNNB1 gene mutation, and intranuclear β-catenin staining positive. Patients with this subtype are typically older, most often have classic medulloblastoma, and have the best clinical prognosis (patients under 16 years of age have better prognosis), with 5-year survival rates exceeding 95% in children and 100% in adults, little tumor dissemination, and often benefit from combination therapy regimens. However, accurate and rapid diagnosis of this subtype is key to effective treatment. Conventional diagnostic methods such as β-catenin immunohistochemical staining, CTNNB1 mutation analysis, and chromosome 6 haploinsufficiency testing have limitations in detecting all cases. In a study of 78 cases of WNT medulloblastoma samples, β-catenin immunohistochemical staining detected only 82% of patients. Combining indicators such as β-catenin immunohistochemical staining (positive) + CTNNB1 mutation (positive) + chromosome 6 (deletion) only detected 77% of WNT medulloblastomas. The remaining patients could show (1) CTNNB1 mutation (positive) + chromosome 6 (deletion) + β-catenin immunohistochemical staining (negative) (8%); (2) CTNNB1 mutation (positive) + chromosome 6 (not deletion) + β-catenin immunohistochemical staining (negative) (8%); (3) only chromosome 6 (no deletion) (5%); (4) lack of any diagnostic indicators (2%). However, unsupervised clustering-based DNA methylation analysis can 100% separate WNT medulloblastoma from other subtypes.

SHH medulloblastoma subtypes account for approximately 25% of all medulloblastomas. While almost all desmoplastic medulloblastomas belong to the SHH subtype, not all SHH medulloblastomas are desmoplastic. SHH medulloblastomas can develop in infants (≤3 years, i-SHH), children/adolescents (3–18 years, p-SHH), and adults (≥18 years, a-SHH) with tumors predominantly located in the cerebellar hemispheres. The prognosis for SHH medulloblastomas is average with less frequent dissemination. The location, histologic type, and clinical prognosis vary by age. For example, 81% of a-SHH occurs in the lateral cerebellar hemisphere, whereas only 67% of p-SHH and 27% of i-SHH occur in this region. Large cell and anaplastic types are common in p-SHH (33%), while desmoplastic and extensive nodular types are common in i-SHH (64%) and a-SHH (51%). The 5-year survival rates for i-SHH, p-SHH, and a-SHH are 80%, 31%, and 52%, respectively. In a 2018 study published in Lancet Oncol, Robinson et al. used methylation to further classify SHH medulloblastomas that occur in infants, children, and adolescents into two subtypes: iSHH-I and iSHH-II. The former subtype had a 5-year progression-free survival rate of 27.8%, while the latter had a rate of 75%. Common mutations in this type include TERT, TP53, PTCH1, SUFU, SMO, N-MYC, Gli2 amplifications, and 17p deletion. In rare cases, a specific mutation, IDH1/IDH2 mutation, can also occur in this type. Group 3 medulloblastoma accounts for about 25% of cases, with a male and younger age predominance, frequent tumor dissemination, and a poor prognosis. This subtype is commonly associated with MYC gene amplification and is often characterized by large cell or classic medulloblastoma histology. However, a recent study published in Cancer Cell by Archer et al. suggested that inhibition of the DNA-activated protein kinase catalytic subunit peptide (PRKDC) could improve the sensitivity of medulloblastomas with MYC gene amplification to radiotherapy. The Group 4 subtype of medulloblastoma represents 35% of all cases and is the most common molecular subtype. While demographically similar to Group 3, it has a relatively good prognosis. The main molecular characteristics of Group 4 subtype are the tetraploid and i(17q) isobaric chromosomes, as well as common amplifications of N-MYC and CDK6. However, compared to glioma, the molecular classification of medulloblastoma remains unclear, especially for Group 3 and Group 4 subtypes, which account for a significant proportion of cases. Despite a lack of clear molecular features for these subtypes, recent research by Lin et al. in Nature (2016) sheds light on Group 4 subtype. Their findings suggest that Lmx1A is a key regulator of Group 4 subtype, driving the differentiation of neural stem cells in the superior rhombomere region of the cerebellum to Group 4 medulloblastoma. In 2018, Gómez et al. published a method in Clin Cancer Res for the rapid differentiation of Group 3 and Group 4 subtypes of medulloblastoma based on methylation characteristics with an accuracy of 92%. Building upon these findings, Goschzik et al. conducted risk stratification for medulloblastoma in Lancet Oncol, 2018, categorizing cases into WNT type, SHH type, and non-WNT/non-SHH type, and guiding treatment accordingly. In WNT type, age is a critical factor that affects prognosis, with patients under 16 years of age having a better prognosis. In SHH type, patients with TP53 mutation or chromosome 17p deletion tend to have a poor prognosis and are more prone to recurrence. Non-WNT/non-SHH type is characterized by a variety of chromosomal ploidy and chromosomal variants. Subgroups with chromosome 7 acquisition, chromosome 8 deletion, and chromosome 11 deletion are considered low-risk groups. Therefore, children aged less than 16 years with WNT type, those with TP53 wild SHH type, and those with non-WNT/non-SHH type with chromosomal variant signatures are in the low clinical risk group and can be considered for relatively conservative treatment. However, those with high-risk medulloblastoma should receive intensive treatment to achieve better outcomes.

In 2019, Sharma et al. conducted a comprehensive analysis based on DNA methylation data from 1501 medulloblastoma cases in Acta Neuropathol and classified Group 3 and Group 4 medulloblastoma into eight subtypes, each with distinct genetic features. Subgroup I had OTX2 amplification in 20% of patients, subgroup II had MYC amplification in 23% of patients, subgroup IV had MYC amplification in 10% of patients, and 21% of patients had MYCN amplification. The eight subtypes were divided into three risk groups based on prognosis. The very high-risk group (5-year overall survival rate was 50%) included subgroup II (often with MYC amplification, 5-year overall survival rate was 50%), subgroup III (often with MYC amplification, 5-year overall survival rate was 43%), and subgroup V (often with MYC/MYCN amplification, 5-year overall survival rate was 59%). The medium-risk group included subgroup VIII, with 35% of patients dying at 5 years after diagnosis. The low-risk group (5-year overall survival rate was 82%) included subgroup I (5-year overall survival rate was 77%), subgroup IV (5-year overall survival rate was 80%), subgroup VI (5-year overall survival rate was 81%), and subgroup VII (5-year overall survival rate was 85%).

Molecular biology is one way to predict the subtype of medulloblastoma, but differences in the biological characteristics of each subtype can also be observed through imaging, providing an important tool for indirectly predicting the subtype. For example, WNT type often occurs in the pontocerebellar region, SHH type often occurs in the lateral cerebellar hemisphere, Group 4 often shows mild enhancement, and Group 3 often exhibits spinal cord metastasis.

At the same time, similar to the spatiotemporal variability in the genetic background of gliomas, different genomic features exist for primary recurrence and primary foci-metastases.

In 2016, Morrissy et al. published a study in Nature that found that the genetic information of primary medulloblastoma tumors in mouse models was significantly different from that of recurrent tumors. Specifically, less than 5% of the genetic information overlapped between the primary and recurrent tumors across the entire genome. Similar conclusions were drawn from analyzing 33 pairs of primary and recurrent human tissue samples during the same period, with less than 12% of the genetic information overlapping between the two types of tumors. One potential explanation for tumor recurrence after treatment is the activation of treatment-resistant signaling pathways. However, these are currently only hypotheses, and further investigation is needed to identify clear mechanisms of action and more specific drivers of recurrence. There are also two key challenges in this process. Firstly, molecular classification of medulloblastoma requires whole-genome sequencing of the tumor, which can be expensive and time-consuming, making it difficult to apply in clinical settings. Secondly, for individuals categorized based on molecular classification, chemotherapy must be validated in additional clinical trials. Nonetheless, the molecular classification of medulloblastoma is an important area of development for the future.

Age is a significant factor in both the diagnosis and prognosis of medulloblastoma. The Huashan neurosurgical team conducted a study on a cohort of 99 adult medulloblastoma cases and found that the proportions of the four molecular subgroups differed slightly from those observed in pediatric cases. Specifically, the SHH subgroup accounted for 50% of cases, followed by Group 4 (18%), WNT (19%), and Group 3 (13%). However, unlike in pediatric cases, molecular subgrouping did not have a significant prognostic impact in the adult cohort. Instead, the study identified KMT2C mutation, histological types, and metastasis as independent prognostic factors in adult medulloblastoma patients. These findings underscore the importance of distinguishing between pediatric and adult medulloblastoma patients when making diagnoses and treatment decisions.

2.7 Molecular Classification of Ependymoma

Ependymoma is a rare type of central nervous system tumor that accounts for 2.1% of primary intracranial tumors and can occur in the supratentorial, infratentorial, or spinal cord regions. Spinal cord ependymomas are most common in adults, while approximately 90% of ependymomas in children occur intracranially, with two-thirds of those originating in the infratentorial region. According to data from other countries, the 10-year survival rate for ependymoma in children is approximately 64%, and in adults, it is around 70%. However, the prognosis for neonates with ependymoma is significantly worse, with a 5-year survival rate ranging from 42 to 55%. The field of ependymoma treatment has seen relatively slow progress in the last decade. Currently, the main treatment options involve surgical resection, with or without radiotherapy, but patient responses to treatment can vary widely, and prognosis is not accurately determined using conventional pathological diagnosis. The rapid development of genomics in recent years has created promising opportunities for the diagnosis and treatment of ependymoma. According to the WHO classification, ependymomas can be divided into WHO grade I subependymoma and myxopapillary ependymoma, WHO grade II ependymomas, and WHO grade III anaplastic ependymoma, with WHO grade II ependymomas being the most common. These tumors can be further divided into four pathological subtypes: cellular, clear cell, papillary, and tanycytic. However, these subtypes are subjective and imprecise, which limits their usefulness in clinical practice. In addition, several rare types of ependymoma have been identified in recent years, including ependymoma with vacuolated cells and ependymoma with adipocytic differentiation.

The Collaborative Ependymoma Research Network (CERN) has been established to advance research on ependymoma, similar to the effort made for medulloblastoma. In 2012, CERN conducted genomic sequencing for 56 cases of infratentorial ependymomas, resulting in the identification of 10 differentially expressed genes: MMP9, TOP2A, TKTL1, COL3A1, LAMB1, COL4A2, TGFBI, GRIA1, SLC14A1, and F5. Based on these genes, infratentorial ependymomas were classified into Group 1 and Group 2. Group 1 patients were mostly WHO grade III tumors and younger in age, while Group 2 patients were predominantly male. The expression levels of these 10 genes were scored on the meta-gene scale, and patients with scores ≥ -0.5 had better PFS and survival than those with scores < -0.5. In 2015, CERN collaborated with 12 institutions to collect 500 ependymoma specimens from various sites and ages to analyze their methylation and transcriptome levels. The results of this study were published in the journal of Cancer Cell. Tumors were divided into three sites: spinal, supratentorial, and infratentorial, each of which contained three molecular subtypes with unique demographic characteristics, histopathological types, genetic backgrounds, and clinical prognoses. In total, nine genotyped ependymomas were identified (including subgroups for supratentorial, infratentorial, and spinal tumors). The supratentorial group consists of the RELA fusion subgroup (constituting approximately 71% of ST-EPNs) and the YAP1 fusion subgroup (approximately 6% of ST-EPNs). The infratentorial group is classified into two subgroups, A and B. The spinal cord is the NF2 mutant type. The worst prognosis is observed in infratentorial group A and the supratentorial RELA fusion subgroup, as per Table 2.1. The age of the patients is a crucial prognostic factor, and younger children tend to have a poorer prognosis than older children in most cases. One of the subgroups of supratentorial ependymoma (ST-EPNs) is characterized by a chromosome 11q13.1 fragmentation rearrangement that results in the formation of C11orf95 and RELA fusion (ST-EPN-RELA). This group of tumors is included in the new 2016 WHO-CNS tumor classification and occurs in both children and adults. Unfortunately, it has a poor prognosis, with a 10-year progression-free survival rate of less than 20% and a 10-year overall survival rate of less than 50%. Interestingly, there is no significant difference in prognosis between patients with total and near-total resection, which suggests that this type of ependymoma may require more intensive treatment such as surgery combined with radiotherapy. However, future clinical trials will be necessary to verify this hypothesis. The direct detection of RELA fusion in clinical settings can be expensive and burdensome. An alternative potential marker for this subtype is the specific expression of L1CAM through immunohistochemistry. Non-RELA fused ST-EPNs are a highly diverse group, comprising approximately 18% of ST-EPNs and may include Yap1 fusion, Bcor tandem replications, EP300-Bcorl1 fusion, or FoxO1-Stk24 fusion. In cases where the oncogene YAP1 is present as a genetic feature with multiple fusions, the patients are mostly children and have a relatively favorable prognosis. Ependymomas located in the infratentorial/posterior fossa region are classified into two groups, PFEPN-A and PF-EPN-B (groups A and B). Pajtler et al. conducted an in-depth analysis of the transcriptome of PF-EPN-A ependymomas and identified two major subtypes, PFA-1 and PFA-2. Further analysis revealed that PFA-1c often

Table 2.1 Molecular classification of ependymomas and associated features

Location	Molecular pathology	Molecular characteristics	Histopathology	WHO	Clinical characteristic
Supratentorial	SE	None	SE	I	Adults, good prognosis
	EPN-YAP1	YAP1 fusion	(Anaplastic) Ependymoma	II/III	Infants/adolescents, good prognosis
	EPN-RELA	RELA fusion	(Anaplastic) Ependymoma	II/I III	Infants/adolescents, poor prognosis
Infratentorial	SE	None	SE	I	Adults, good prognosis
	EPN-A	None	(Anaplastic) Ependymoma	II/III	Infants/adolescents, poor prognosis
	EPN-B	Chromosome instability	(Anaplastic) Ependymoma	II/III	Infants/adolescents, good prognosis
Spinal cord	SE	6q deletion	SE	I	Adults, good prognosis
	MPE	Chromosome instability	MPE	I	Adults, good prognosis
	EPN	NF2 mutation	(Anaplastic) Ependymoma	II/III	Adults, good prognosis

SE subependymoma, *EPN* ependymoma, *MPE* myxopapillary ependymoma exhibits an increase in chromosome 1q and has a relatively poor prognosis. On the other hand, patients with PFA-2c ependymomas have a 5-year overall survival rate of over 90%. Unlike other ependymomas, PFA-2c tumors express high levels of Otx2, which is a potential biomarker for a subtype of ependymoma with a favorable prognosis. The H3K27M mutation is a significant genetic feature of diffuse midline gliomas and can be found in 4.2% of ependymomas, mainly in PFA-1 types (with PFA-1f being the most prevalent). CXorf67 mutation is present in all subtypes except for PFA-1f. Furthermore, an increase in chromosome arm 1q is observed in PF-EPN-A (PFA-1c), PF-EPN-B, and ST-EPN-RELA subtypes, which is an independent factor contributing to a poorer prognosis. The histomorphology of PFEPN-A and PF-EPN-B groups is comparable, but their clinical prognosis differs. The former primarily occurs in infants and young children, is typically not located in the midline, is challenging to remove entirely, and is linked to a high recurrence rate. The latter is more prevalent in adolescents and young adults and has a comparatively better prognosis. Thus, a prompt and accurate differentiation between the two ependymoma subtypes is crucial for personalized treatment. Although DNA methylation can distinguish between them, it is not practical for routine clinical use. To address this, Panwalkar et al. utilized H3K27me3 immunohistochemical staining as a quick and reliable method of differentiation. Their study demonstrated that H3K27me3 immunohistochemical staining is negative in PF-EPN-A and positive in PF-EPN-B, with a sensitivity of 99% and specificity of 100% when compared to the gold standard methylation index. Additionally, H3K4me3 can differentiate the PF-EPN-A group, and its expression not only impacts the progression-free survival of patients in this group but also increases the sensitivity of ependymoma primary cells to chemotherapy when its expression is reduced. However, as molecules advances, some molecular classifications cannot be accurately categorized into a particular tissue type. Witt et al. conducted a study comparing the histological and molecular classification of 122 cases of ependymoma based on DNA methylation analysis. Their findings demonstrated that the histological and molecular classification of subependymoma were consistent. Moreover, 19 cases with a histological diagnosis of ependymoma (WHO grade II) but with a molecular staging of subependymoma (WHO grade I) and a histology of myxopapillary ependymoma (MPE) were all attributed to the molecular classification of spinal MPE. The molecular classification includes 15 WHO class II histological types, but only 7 molecular subtypes are identified in WHO class II histological types. This indicates that molecular subtyping provides a more complete and comprehensive understanding of patient prognosis than conventional pathological classification and can even guide future treatment for ependymoma.

Several other molecular markers of ependymoma have been identified. For instance, the epithelial growth factor receptor (EGFR) has been proposed as a prognostic indicator for ependymoma. In a study involving 22 patients with WHO grade II and III ependymoma, immunohistochemistry was used to test for EGFR expression. The study found that patients with positive EGFR expression had a shorter overall survival (OS) compared to those with negative expression. Moreover, positive EGFR expression was more common in patients with high-grade ependymoma, indicating a poorer prognosis. This study suggests that EGFR may be a useful prognostic marker for ependymoma, and further analysis found that patients with overexpression of both EGFR and trap protein-1 had significantly shorter OS and PFS. While some studies have found that patients with EGFR-positive ependymomas have a better prognosis, the mechanism and prognostic impact of EGFR in ependymomas require further investigation. Nucleolin, a protein located in the nucleus, has been detected in tumor cells such as hepatocellular carcinoma and prostate cancer, and some studies suggest that ependymomas with nucleolin overexpression have a poor prognosis. Additionally, the

Canadian Pediatric Brain Tumor Center has shown that enhancer of zeste homolog 2 (EZH2) expression clearly affects the prognosis of pediatric ependymoma. However, these studies are limited by small sample sizes and single sites and therefore do not provide a comprehensive understanding of the overall prognosis of ependymoma.

Further Reading

Archer TC, Ehrenberger T, Mundt F, et al. Proteomics, post-translational modifications, and Integrative analyses reveal molecular heterogeneity within medulloblastoma subgroups. Cancer Cell. 2018;34(3):396–410. e8

Chan AK, Shi ZF, Li KK, Wang WW, Chen H, Chung NY, Chan DT, Poon WS, Loong HH, Liu XZ, Zhang ZY, Mao Y, Ng HK. Combinations of single-gene biomarkers can precisely stratify 1028 adult gliomas for prognostication. Front Oncol. 2022;12:839302.

Dasgupta A, Gupta T, Sridhar E, et al. Pediatric patients with SHH medulloblastoma fail differently as compared with adults: possible implications for treatment modifications. J Pediatr Hematol Oncol. 2019;41(8):e499–505.

de Souza CF, Sabedot TS, Malta TM, Stetson L, Morozova O, Sokolov A, Laird PW, Wiznerowicz M, Iavarone A, Snyder J, deCarvalho A, Sanborn Z, McDonald KL, Friedman WA, Tirapelli D, Poisson L, Mikkelsen T, Carlotti CG Jr, Kalkanis S, Zenklusen J, Salama SR, Barnholtz-Sloan JS, Noushmehr H. A distinct DNA methylation shift in a subset of glioma CpG island methylator phenotypes during tumor recurrence. Cell Rep. 2018;23(2):637–51.

Diplas BH, He X, Brosnan-Cashman JA, Liu H, Chen LH, Wang Z, Moure CJ, Killela PJ, Loriaux DB, Lipp ES, Greer PK, Yang R, Rizzo AJ, Rodriguez FJ, Friedman AH, Friedman HS, Wang S, He Y, McLendon RE, Bigner DD, Jiao Y, Waitkus MS, Meeker AK, Yan H. The genomic landscape of TERT promoter wildtype-IDH wildtype glioblastoma. Nat Commun. 2018;9(1):2087.

El-Ayadi M, Egervari K, Merkler D, et al. Concurrent IDH1 and SMARCB1 mutations in pediatric medulloblastoma: a case report. Front Neurol. 2018;9:398.

Fomchenko EI, Erson-Omay EZ, Moliterno J. A novel finding of an IDH2 mutation in an interesting adult Sonic Hedgehog mutated medulloblastoma. J Neurooncol. 2019;144(1):231–3.

Fukuoka K, Kanemura Y, Shofuda T, et al. Significance of molecular classification of ependymomas: C11orf95-RELA fusion-negative supratentorial ependymomas are a heterogeneous group of tumors. Acta Neuropathol Commun. 2018;6(1):134.

Gomez S, Garrido-Garcia A, Garcia-Gerique L, et al. A novel method for rapid molecular subgrouping of medulloblastoma. Clin Cancer Res. 2018;24(6):1355–63.

Goschzik T, Schwalbe EC, Hicks D, et al. Prognostic effect of whole chromosomal aberration signatures in standard-risk, non-WNT/non-SHH medulloblastoma: a retrospective, molecular analysis of the HIT-SIOP PNET 4 trial. Lancet Oncol. 2018;19(12):1602–16.

Korshunov A, Sahm F, Zheludkova O, et al. DNA methylation profiling is a method of choice for molecular verification of pediatric WNT-activated medulloblastomas. Neuro Oncol. 2019;21(2):214–21.

Li KK, Shi ZF, Malta TM, Chan AK, Cheng S, Kwan JSH, Yang RR, Poon WS, Mao Y, Noushmehr H, Chen H, Ng HK. Identification of subsets of IDH-mutant glioblastomas with distinct epigenetic and copy number alterations and stratified clinical risks. Neurooncol Adv. 2019;1(1):vdz015.

Mata-Mbemba D, Zapotocky M, Laughlin S, et al. MRI characteristics of primary tumors and metastatic lesions in molecular subgroups of pediatric medulloblastoma: a single-center study. AJNR Am J Neuroradiol. 2018;39(5):949–55.

Pagès M, Pajtler KW, Puget S, et al. Diagnostics of pediatric supratentorial RELA ependymomas: integration of information from histopathology, genetics, DNA methylation and imaging. Brain Pathol. 2019;29(3):325–35.

Pajtler KW, Wen J, Sill M, et al. Molecular heterogeneity and CXorf67 alterations in posterior fossa group A (PFA) ependymomas. Acta Neuropathol. 2018;136(2):211–26.

Panwalkar P, Clark J, Ramaswamy V, et al. Immunohistochemical analysis of H3K27me3 demonstrates global reduction in group-A childhood posterior fossa ependymoma and is a powerful predictor of outcome. Acta Neuropathol. 2017;134(5):705–14.

Robinson GW, Rudneva VA, Buchhalter I, et al. Risk-adapted therapy for young children with medulloblastoma (SJYC07): therapeutic and molecular outcomes from a multicentre, phase 2 trial. Lancet Oncol. 2018;19(6):768–84.

Ruda R, Reifenberger G, Frappaz D, et al. EANO guidelines for the diagnosis and treatment of ependymal tumors. Neuro Oncol. 2018;20(4):445–56.

Sharma T, Schwalbe EC, Williamson D, et al. Second-generation molecular subgrouping of medulloblastoma: an international meta-analysis of Group 3 and Group 4 subtypes. Acta Neuropathol. 2019;138(2):309–26.

Witt H, Gramatzki D, Hentschel B, et al. DNA methylation-based classification of ependymomas in adulthood: implications for diagnosis and treatment. Neuro Oncol. 2018;20(12):1616–24.

Wong GC, Li KK, Wang WW, Liu AP, Huang QJ, Chan AK, Poon MF, Chung NY, Wong QH, Chen H, Chan DTM, Liu XZ, Mao Y, Zhang ZY, Shi ZF, Ng HK. Clinical and mutational profiles of adult medulloblastoma groups. Acta Neuropathol Commun. 2020;8(1):191.

Wong QH, Li KK, Wang WW, Malta TM, Noushmehr H, Grabovska Y, Jones C, Chan AK, Kwan JS, Huang QJ, Wong GC, Li WC, Liu XZ, Chen H, Chan DT, Mao Y, Zhang ZY, Shi ZF, Ng HK. Molecular landscape of IDH-mutant primary astrocytoma Grade IV/glioblastomas. Mod Pathol. 2021;34(7):1245–60.

3 Liquid Biopsy in the Future of Glioma Diagnosis and Treatment Occupies a Key Position

Wei Hua, Wei Zhu, and Ruofan Huang

Liquid biopsy has emerged as a promising technology in the field of oncology in recent years. Tumors, including gliomas, release soluble substances into various body fluids, such as blood, cerebrospinal fluid, and urine, which can provide insights into the characteristics of the tumor. The journal MIT Technology Review listed liquid biopsy of malignant tumors as one of the top ten breakthrough technologies in 2015, as it allows for rapid and simple screening for most tumors. While liquid biopsy is primarily based on a simple blood test, it can also be extended to other body fluids, such as cerebrospinal fluid and urine. This enables the monitoring of tumor changes repeatedly and dynamically, as well as the establishment of gene expression profiles of tumors. Additionally, liquid biopsy can guide targeted drug therapy and predict efficacy, making it possible to develop individualized treatment strategies in real-time. Compared to surgical or puncture biopsies, liquid biopsy is a complementary technique that provides a less invasive and more convenient method of obtaining tumor samples for analysis.

In recent years, circulating tumor cells (CTCs) have emerged as a promising new biomarker in oncology research, including in the detection of glioblastoma (GBM). CTCs are cells shed by proliferating or inactivated tumor cells into the surrounding body fluids, including the circulatory system, which can lead to metastasis and the formation of CTCs in distant sites. In addition to CTCs, circulating tumor DNA (ctDNA) is another type of biomarker that is released by tumor cells into the surrounding microenvironment and body fluids, including blood. Furthermore, recent research has focused on the use of extracellular vesicles, particularly exosomes, as carriers to transport free molecules such as miRNA and protect them from short-term degradation. Current liquid biopsy technology primarily targets CTCs and ctDNA. However, detecting these biomarkers in early-stage tumors can be challenging due to the low amounts present in the circulation. Nevertheless, advances in detection technology have led to improvements in the sensitivity and specificity of liquid biopsy, while reducing costs and increasing clinical applicability. Proteomic methods can detect proteins in the circulatory system, and commercial kits can isolate free DNA (cfDNA) and miRNA in serum. Extracellular vesicles have also emerged as a promising target for liquid biopsy, as they offer greater stability than other RNAs.

Tumor markers are substances that are produced specifically by malignant tumors or in response to tumor stimulation and are typically detected in body fluids such as blood, cerebrospinal fluid, plasma fluid, and urine. They can provide valuable information for the early diagnosis,

W. Hua · W. Zhu · R. Huang (✉)
Department of Neurosurgery, Huashan Hospital, Fudan University, Shanghai, China
e-mail: ruofanhung@fudan.edu.cn

Y. Mao (ed.), *Progress in the Diagnosis and Treatment of Gliomas*, Experts' Perspectives on Medical Advances, https://doi.org/10.1007/978-981-99-0123-4_3

classification, prognosis, and guidance of treatment for tumors and can be tested using immunological and biochemical methods. The discovery of tumor markers dates back to 1845, when Bence-Jones observed elevated levels of a protein in the urine of myeloma patients. Since then, numerous hormones, isoenzymes, and proteins have been found to be altered in patients with tumors, such as human chorionic gonadotropin (HCG), which was identified as a marker for choriocarcinoma by Zondek. Other embryonic protein markers, such as AFP and CEA, were also discovered in subsequent years. The invention of monoclonal antibodies (McAbs) in 1975 further advanced the field of tumor marker detection, and the use of tumor markers in clinical practice was formally introduced at the British Conference on Oncogenesis Biology and Medicine in 1979. In recent years, a multitude of new tumor markers have been discovered, driving advancements in tumor diagnosis and treatment. However, identifying specific markers for gliomas, particularly high-grade gliomas (HGG), remains a significant challenge.

3.1 Blood Liquid Biopsy in the Diagnosis and Treatment of Glioma

Blood liquid biopsy in particular has advantages in terms of accessibility and convenience. However, there are challenges to overcome, such as potential interference from other organs in the blood circulation, which may affect the accuracy of liquid biopsy results. Moreover, the blood–brain barrier can prevent the detection of some important proteins, limiting the application of liquid biopsy in brain tumors such as gliomas. Despite these challenges, progress has been made in the detection of serum tumor-associated proteins for various types of cancer. Xu et al. conducted a proteomic analysis and discovered changes in several proteins, including α2-macroglobulin, CA199, factor VII, macrophage chemokines, and stem cell factors, in the plasma of glioma patients. They also found that plasma MIP-α levels reflect glioma hyperplasia and that TIMP1 levels are elevated in the plasma of GBM patients. However, peripheral blood testing for glioma markers is still developing slowly due to its low sensitivity and specificity. With advances in biotechnology, peripheral blood testing may have a role in predicting malignant glioma recurrence and the effectiveness of antitumor drugs. The glioma team at our hospital used ELISA and 2D western blot to detect GFAP in blood and found that 25% of glioma patients had increased expression of GFAP in plasma, which correlated with tumor grade.

Serum proteomics studies of GBM are currently in the process of development. In a recent study based on surface-enhanced spectroscopy, CXCR4, S100A8, and S100A9 were found to be promising, but further validation of the findings is needed. Other studies have proposed completely different protein profiles, such as bead-binding proteins and thyroid hormone-binding proteins. However, a comparison of serum levels of GFAP, S100, NSE, and β-synuclein in patients with different grades of glioma and healthy subjects using electrochemical fluorescence did not reveal significant differences. IDH1 and IDH2 mutations have been a point of interest in the serological detection of glioma. However, the levels of their metabolite 2-hydroxyglutaric acid (2-HG) in serum have not shown correlation with IDH1/IDH2 mutation status or tumor size. The protein EGFRv III is specific to glioma and expressed in some patients. It can be detected in exosomes and may serve as a biomarker for EGFRv III-targeted therapy. If changes in EGFRv III in tumor tissue of glioma patients treated with EGFRv III vaccine can be reflected in serology in the future, it may become more widely used. VEGF plays a crucial role in glioma vascularization and malignant progression, and some studies have suggested that VEGF levels in glioma patients are proportional to tumor vascular density. However, further research has failed to confirm its role in the diagnosis and assessment of glioma outcomes.

The length of ctDNA ranges from 150 to 200 bp, and it has been shown that it can reflect various types of mutations such as point mutations and amplifications in many types of tumors, including gliomas. Thus, ctDNA is a specific tumor biomarker that can be characterized, quantified, and tracked. In patients with solid tumors, including gliomas, ctDNA has been detected, and common glioma mutations such as IDH1, EGFRv III, MGMT methylation, and 1p19q heterozygous can be identified. Compared to circulating tumor cells (CTCs), ctDNA appears to be more abundant and was found in 13 out of 16 patients without detectable CTCs. The cellular detection threshold for ctDNA is approximately 50×10^6, which is much lower than the cellular level visible on imaging. While the half-life of ctDNA in serum is not yet known, a study found that the half-life of EBV DNA in patients with nasopharyngeal carcinoma was less than 3 h, suggesting that the dynamics of ctDNA may reflect real-time tumor homeostasis. This finding indicates that dynamic changes in ctDNA may reflect intratumor homeostasis in real time. The high sensitivity and dynamic changes of ctDNA, coupled with the rapid development of various assay technologies, may facilitate rapid biopsy of serum specimens.

miRNAs are small non-coding RNA molecules consisting of 21–24 nucleotides. Since their discovery in 2000, over 2000 miRNAs have been identified to play crucial roles in regulating both normal and tumor cells. Due to their roles in oncogenesis, anti-oncogenesis, and intercellular signaling, miRNAs are regarded as the most promising molecules in extracellular vesicles (EVs) for tumor diagnosis and prognosis. miRNAs are known to reflect tissue-specific "fingerprints," and the miRNA profiles in exosomes of metastatic tumors are consistent with those of primary lesions. Clinical trials are underway to investigate the role of miRNAs in assessing the outcomes of kidney and lung cancer. miRNAs in GBM tumor tissues have also been studied to predict prognosis and treatment response, and subtype-specific miRNA profiles can be utilized for survival prediction. A retrospective analysis based on the TCGA database revealed a positive correlation between miR-130a and TMZ efficacy, independent of MGMT methylation status. MiR-21 is the most widely studied miRNA in glioma, and meta-analysis demonstrated that it is a reliable soluble biomarker for glioma diagnosis that can distinguish and exclude pseudoprogression and radionecrosis. Therefore, miR-21 is considered a potential therapeutic target.

CTCs can be utilized for early diagnosis of metastatic disease and monitoring of recurrence. This is particularly important when tumor biopsy is not feasible. CTCs offer a comprehensive reflection of tumor characteristics, and even a single CTC can be used for genomic analysis. However, their accuracy for GBM is questionable as GBM is a highly heterogeneous tumor. In the past, it was believed that CTCs were not present in glioma patients due to the blood–brain barrier. Nevertheless, in recent years, extracranial metastases from gliomas have been occasionally reported, and several groups have detected CTCs in GBM patients using various methods.

In a separate investigation, CTCs were identified using GFAP in only 20% of the 141 cases of peripheral blood mononuclear cells. With the advent of single-cell genome sequencing, specific mutations that match the primary tumor can be discovered in CTCs, providing a glimpse into the tumor's genetic profile. Single markers such as GFAP, telomerase, or other markers do not capture the accurate frequency or heterogeneity of CTCs. Therefore, the integration of multiple technologies or markers will be required to integrate CTCs into routine clinical diagnosis in the future, as well as to track cell subtypes during treatment. The primary challenge limiting the widespread application of CTCs is their paucity. In many patients, only a few CTCs can be detected in 10 mL of peripheral blood, making it too difficult to evaluate efficacy using so few CTCs. Additionally, the relationship between CTCs and tumor stem cells is intriguing. A small percentage of breast cancer CTCs display stem cell markers, which are frequently discovered in metastatic cases and frequently indicate poor prognosis. Further study is required to determine whether CTCs are closely connected to stem cells in gliomas.

3.2 The Use of Cerebrospinal Fluid (CSF) Biopsy Has Emerged as a New Area of Focus in Research on Glioma Diagnosis and Treatment

CSF testing offers unique advantages for the diagnosis and treatment of central nervous system (CNS) disorders. Produced by the choroid plexus, CSF circulates in the ventricles, subarachnoid space, and central canal of the spinal cord, playing a crucial role in nourishing brain cells, metabolite transport, acid-base balance regulation, intracranial pressure balancing, and brain temperature maintenance. Despite being similar to plasma and lymphatic fluid in nature, CSF lacks bilirubin, fibrinogen, complement, antibody, and cholesterol. As CSF is exclusively produced in the central nervous system, it has a clean background, which enhances its specificity for the diagnosis of CNS diseases. Various molecular markers in CSF have been linked to Parkinson's disease, dementia, multiple sclerosis, and amyotrophic (spinal) lateral sclerosis. Moreover, several studies have explored the use of CSF in glioma patients to detect different indicators, with the aim of enabling early diagnosis and monitoring of relapse.

A metabolomics study of glioma patients analyzed their CSF and found significant increases in metabolites such as lactate and citrate in GBM patients with IDH1 mutations, with levels associated with prognosis. Our neurosurgery glioma team conducted a systematic review of glioma CSF proteomics and found 19 proteins with significant changes in either CSF or tumor capsule fluid, with WNT4, GAL, IL-6, and HSPA5 differing among grades. We demonstrated that IL-6 was significantly increased in glioma CSF, and we also investigated B7H1 and B7H3 in CSF, finding that both were significantly higher in glioma patients than in normal subjects and were positively correlated with primary tumor expression.

The content of miR-21 in the CSF of GBM patients was almost ten times higher than that of normal individuals, and it was predominantly found in EVs. However, after complete tumor resection, the miR-21 content in the CSF was only 1/50 of the pre-surgery level. A total of 58 types of miRNA were identified in CSF, and levels of miR-23 and miR-150 were significantly elevated compared to normal levels. Therefore, identifying exosome-specific miRNAs in CSF is a potential novel method for glioma diagnosis. In a study by Mattos Arruda, specific ctDNA was compared in the CSF and plasma of 12 brain tumor patients with IDH1 (R132H), TP53 (R114C), and ANK2 (K2337X) mutations using massively parallel sequencing. It was found that CSF was more sensitive in predicting tumor progression and treatment response.

3.3 Urine Liquid Biopsy May Be a New Idea for Glioma Diagnosis and Treatment

Efforts to detect relevant proteins in urine for glioma diagnosis have been ongoing for a while, with limited progress. In 2015, a study was published investigating the detection of 2-hydroxyglutarate (2-HG) in the serum and urine of glioma patients. 2-HG is a small metabolite that can be detected in various body fluids. The study demonstrated that 2-HG in urine can be quickly, easily, and noninvasively detected using tandem mass spectrometry (MS/MS) or high-performance liquid chromatography (HPLC). The mean serum concentrations of 2-HG in patients with wild-type and mutant IDH were not significantly different, but there was a significant difference in urinary levels of 2-HG, with the concentration in wild-type patients being significantly higher than that in mutant patients. The serum/urine ratio of 2-HG was also significantly different, with the ratio in mutant patients being higher than that in wild-type patients. Both tests suggest that urine 2-HG can be used for the preliminary determination of IDH mutation in patients. In addition, it has been observed that in other tumors with IDH mutations, urine 2-HG levels significantly decrease after tumor resection, indicating that urine 2-HG is a potential indicator for prognostic evaluation.

Screening specific markers for gliomas is a challenging task due to their heterogeneity. While cerebrospinal fluid and urine have their advantages and disadvantages as sources of liquid biopsy, they may not be sufficient to accurately reflect the tumor grade. Thus, liquid biopsy cannot replace conventional pathology in diagnosis and treatment strategies. Nonetheless, with the advancement of technology and increasing focus on malignancy research, significant progress has been made in glioma research. However, the search for glioma-specific markers is still ongoing. Next-generation sequencing and research related to various tumor omics fingerprints and profiles are expected to help identify multiple indicators for liquid biopsy diagnosis in the future, such as radiomics combined with liquid biopsy. These liquid biopsy technologies may optimize glioma treatment by providing minimally invasive, individualized, and real-time diagnosis.

Further Reading

Akers JC, Ramakrishnan V, Kim R, et al. MiR-21 in the extracellular vesicles (EVs) of cerebrospinal fluid (CSF): a platform for glioblastoma biomarker development. PLoS One. 2013;8(10):e78115.

Areeb Z, Stylli SS, Koldej R, et al. MicroRNA as potential biomarkers in glioblastoma. J Neurooncol. 2015;125(2):237–48.

Bettegowda C, Sausen M, Leary RJ, et al. Detection of circulating tumor DNA in early- and late-stage human malignancies. Sci Transl Med. 2014;6(224): 224ra24.

Chen H, Li X, Li W, et al. miR-130a can predict response to temozolomide in patients with glioblastoma multiforme, independently of O6-methylguanine-DNA methyltransferase. J Transl Med. 2015;13:69.

Chistiakov DA, Chekhonin VP. Extracellular vesicles shed by glioma cells: pathogenic role and clinical value. Tumour Biol. 2014;35(9):8425–38.

DeMattos-Arruda L, Mayor R, Ng CK, et al. Cerebrospinal fluid-derived circulating tumour DNA better represents the genomic alterations of brain tumours than plasma. Nat Commun. 2015;6:8839.

Godlewski J, Krichevsky AM, Johnson MD, et al. Belonging to a network-microRNAs, extracellular vesicles, and the glioblastoma microenvironment. Neuro Oncol. 2015;17(5):652–62.

Heitzer E, Auer M, Ulz P, et al. Circulating tumor cells and DNA as liquid biopsies. Genome Med. 2013;5(8):73.

Lange RP, Everett A, Dulloor P, et al. Evaluation of eight plasma proteins as candidate blood-based biomarkers for malignant gliomas. Cancer Invest. 2014;32(8):423–9.

Lebofsky R, Decraene C, Bernard V, et al. Circulating tumor DNA as anon-invasive substitute to metastasis biopsy for tumor genotyping and personalized medicine in a prospective trial across all tumor types. Mol Oncol. 2015;9(4):783–90.

Li L, Paz AC, Wilky BA, et al. Treatment with a small molecule mutant IDH1 inhibitor suppresses tumorigenic activity and decreases production of the oncometabolite 2-hydroxyglutarate in human chondrosarcoma cells. PLoS One. 2015;10(9):e0133813.

Lombardi G, Corona G, Bellu L, et al. Diagnostic value of plasma and urinary 2-hydroxyglutarate to identify patients with isocitrate dehydrogenase-mutated glioma. Oncologist. 2015;20(5):562–7.

MacArthur KM, Kao GD, Chandrasekaran S, et al. Detection of brain tumor cells in the peripheral blood by a telomerase promoter-based assay. Cancer Res. 2014;74(8):2152–9.

Mikaelian I, Scicchitano M, Mendes O, et al. Frontiers in preclinical safety biomarkers: microRNAs and messenger RNAs. Toxicol Pathol. 2013;41(1):18–31.

Mimeault M, Batras K. Molecular biomarkers of cancer stem/progenitor cells associated with progression, metastases, and treatment resistance of aggressive cancers. Cancer Epidemiol Biomark Prev. 2014;23(2):234–54.

Müller C, Holtschmidt J, Auer M, et al. Hematogenous dissemination of glioblastoma multiforme. Sci Transl Med. 2014;6(247):247ra101.

Popescu ID, Codrici E, Albulescu L, et al. Potential serum biomarkers for glioblastoma diagnostic assessed by proteomic approaches. Proteome Sci. 2014;12(1):47.

Qu S, Guan J, Liu Y. Identification of microRNAs as novel biomarkers for glioma detection: a meta-analysis based on 11 articles. J Neurol Sci. 2015;348(1/2):181–7.

Schuster J, Lai RK, Rechtl D, et al. A phase II, multicenter trial of rindopepimut (CDX-110) in newly diagnosed glioblastoma: the ACT III study. Neuro Oncol. 2015;17(6):854–61.

Advances in Glioma Stem Cell Research

4

Wei Hua and Hui Yang

Glioma stem cells (GSCs) are a self-renewing subpopulation of glioma cells with high tumorigenicity, self-renewal ability, and resistance to radiotherapy. They are thought to be a key factor in glioma recurrence, also known as glioma-initiating cells (GICs).

4.1 Glioma Stem Cells Are Closely Related to Neural Stem Cells

Bonnet first identified the presence of tumor stem cells in acute myeloid leukemia (AML). They isolated a subset of cells that were able to induce AML in immunodeficient mice and found that these cells expressed similar cell surface markers to hematopoietic stem cells. The AML originating from these cells had similar biological properties to the primary tumor. CD44+ CD24− cells were isolated from breast cancer and identified as tumor stem cells, demonstrating that stem cells also exist in solid tumors.

Several groups have identified GSCs in gliomas based on neural stem cell (NSC), such as their ability to form neurosphere-like structures in suspension under in vitro experimental neural stem cell culture conditions (no serum, no cell adhesion, epidermal growth factor, fibroblast growth factor, etc.) along with self-renewal and differentiation abilities. Since then, several markers associated with GSCs have been identified, among which CD133, also known as Prominin-1, is the most important and acts as a cell surface receptor. Singh et al. have shown that CD133+ glioma cells are tumorigenic in immunodeficient mice and can form tumors with morphological features and marker molecules similar to the primary tumor, while CD133− cells do not. However, recent studies have also shown that CD133− cells have self-renewal capabilities and induce tumors. As a result, researchers are still searching for more specific markers of GSCs. Currently, the most commonly used markers of GSCs include broad-spectrum stem cell markers (CD133), neural stem cell markers (A2B5, Nestin), embryonic stem cell markers (Sox, Nanog), and cell adhesion molecules (CD15, CD44, L1CAM). The main characteristics of GSCs can be summarized as self-renewal, tumorigenicity, expression of stem cell markers, and multi-directional differentiation potential.

There are two main differences between GSCs and NSCs. Firstly, GSCs are more self-renewing and can maintain their self-renewal ability in a serum-containing culture medium. Secondly, cells differentiated from GSCs express tubulin-III and GFAP, while the simultaneous expression of different lineage markers is rare in cells differentiated from NSCs.

W. Hua · H. Yang (✉)
Department of Neurosurgery, Huashan Hospital, Fudan University, Shanghai, China
e-mail: hui_yang@fudan.edu.cn

Y. Mao (ed.), *Progress in the Diagnosis and Treatment of Gliomas*, Experts' Perspectives on Medical Advances, https://doi.org/10.1007/978-981-99-0123-4_4

Also, two main hypotheses about the origin of GSCs were reported. The first hypothesis suggests that GSCs originate from neural stem cells, which have very similar molecular characteristics and biological properties. The subventricular zone of the brain is the main area where neural stem cells exist; it has been found that the development of glioblastoma is closely related to the subventricular zone. The probability of tumors in Nestin-positive cells was significantly higher than that in GFAP-positive cells. The above studies suggest that GSCs are derived from the malignant transformation of neural stem cells. The second hypothesis proposes that progenitor cells or mature astrocytes can reactivate the pathways regulating self-renewal through gene mutations and genetic trait changes, thereby increasing the ability of self-renewal and tumor formation. However, this hypothesis does not fully explain the origin of GSCs, and further investigation is needed in the future.

4.2 Glioma Stem Cells Have Treatment-Resistant Biology

GSCs exhibit typical stem cells characteristics, such as self-renewal, proliferation, and multidirectional differentiation potential, and CD133+ cells can continuously proliferate on stem cell medium to form suspended, smooth tumor cell spheres, while in normal serum, the peripheral cells develop protrusions and extend radially in all directions, and these cells can express neuronal and glial markers. In addition, GSCs, like normal stem cells, can create a microenvironment (stem cell niche) suitable for their survival and immune escape by secreting cellular factors and chemokines.

Radiotherapy is an essential treatment for glioma, and as research progresses, GSCs have been found to be a significant cause of resistance to radiotherapy. After radiation treatment, CD133+ cells formed significantly larger colonies and tumors than CD133− cells. The former activated DNA damage repair mechanisms more efficiently, indicating that GSCs may escape radiotherapy by initiating repair mechanisms, including prolonging the cell cycle and expressing CHK kinase. It has also been demonstrated that radiotherapy promotes autophagy in GSCs after inhibiting DNA-dependent kinases. Radiotherapy may also promote converting tumor cells to GSCs, leading to a vicious cycle of GSC resistance to radiotherapy. GSCs have been shown to have enhanced DNA damage repair mechanisms compared to non-stem cancer cells, which may contribute to their resistance to standard therapies. One study published in Neuro-Oncology in 2018 investigated the DNA damage repair mechanisms in GSCs and found that they had increased activity of the base excision repair pathway, which is responsible for repairing single-stranded DNA breaks. Additionally, GSCs were found to have a higher expression of DNA repair proteins, such as PARP1 and XRCC1, than non-stem cancer cells. The study also identified a subset of GSCs with mutations in DNA damage repair genes, such as ATM and CHEK2, which may contribute to their increased DNA repair capacity. Another study published in Cell Reports in 2019 investigated the role of the DNA damage response protein, RAD52 in GSCs. The study found that RAD52 was highly expressed in GSCs compared to non-stem cancer cells and was required to repair DNA double-strand breaks in GSCs. The study also demonstrated that targeting RAD52 with a small molecule inhibitor sensitized GSCs to radiation therapy.

Similarly, many gliomas relapse after chemotherapy and acquire multidrug resistance, with GSCs identified as the surviving drug-resistant cells after chemotherapy. Comparative analysis of CD133+ and CD133− cells isolated from glioma specimens revealed that the expression of the ABC superfamily of multi-drug resistance proteins (MDR1 and MDR2) was much higher in the former than in the latter, suggesting that GSCs are the surviving drug-resistant cells after chemotherapy. After TMZ treatment of gliomas, GSCs originating from the subventricular zone dominate tumor recurrence, and targeted intervention of these stem cells significantly retards tumor growth. Recently, there have been many studies on the mechanism of drug resistance. Inhibition of Notch and Shh pathways significantly increased the responsiveness of GSCs to TMZ, and the same effect was achieved by reducing the expression of TAp73 and mGluR genes. Bian Xiuwu's team found that GSCs have a high level and activity of RTK, BMX, which leads to the destructive growth of tumor stem cells in the brain, while BMX is almost absent in normal neural stem cells in the brain, suggesting that BMX is a specific therapeutic target for glioma tumor stem cells. They found that applying Ibrutinib specifically killed GSCs and synergized with conventional radiation therapy to improve antitumor efficacy.

Immune escape is also an important reason why GSCs are resistant to available therapies. It is believed that GSCs promote tumor immune escape in three ways: first, by activating abnormal immune cells such as regulatory T cells (Treg); second, by expressing negative co-stimulatory molecules such as MHC I, B7-H1, and B7-H4 on their surface, and GSCs can also upregulate B7-H4 expression in microglia through the IL-6/STAT-3 pathway, thus acting indirectly through immune-negative microglia; third, by secreting immunosuppressive factors such as TGF-β, PGE2, CCL2, and galectin-3.

Given the important role of GSCs in drug resistance and treatment resistance in glioma, treatments targeting GSCs are expected to be more effective in suppressing glioma. Immunotherapies targeting GSCs have been developed, with stem cell-like antigens found to be more antigenic than conventional antigens. Phase I clinical trials of stem cell-like antigen-sensitized dendritic cell (DC) vaccines have demonstrated that they are safe and feasible for glioma patients. Combined with chemotherapy, it could prolong survival.

4.3 Activation of Different Signal Transduction Mechanisms Plays an Important Role in Glioma Stem Cells

With the rapid development of molecular biology, there is an increasing number of studies on the signaling pathways of GSCs, which can better explain their biological behavior and guide treatment. The main signal transduction involves the following three aspects.

4.3.1 Extracellular to Intracellular Transduction

The behavior of GSCs is easily influenced by extracellular signals that act through a ligand-receptor mechanism on the cell surface to activate downstream signaling pathways to initiate cascade reactions and play subsequent biological roles. However, for the maintenance of GSCs, we have selected the most important pathways—Shh, Wnt, Notch, TGF-β, and RTK pathways—briefly described here.

The Shh signaling pathway: Shh binds to its receptor and activates a set of transduction molecules called Gli, which activate or inhibit downstream targets by translocating to the nucleus. Shh is essential for self-renewal and tumorigenesis of GSCs, and Shh inhibitors can reduce tumor proliferation and promote apoptosis. Inhibition of the Shh pathway has been found to amplify the tumor-killing effect of TMZ, and in vivo tests have also shown that it can block the growth of GSCs. Some studies have also demonstrated that Shh inhibitors can hinder the growth of GSCs, preventing them from becoming tumors in vivo. Still, they have found that Shh inhibitors can increase the survival rate of GSCs after radiotherapy. The synergistic effect of this pathway with Gli1 has also received much attention in recent years. In summary, the Shh pathway is important for GSCs, and its inhibitors may improve the efficacy of conventional therapies.

Notch signaling pathway: Notch protein is a single transmembrane receptor that mediates cellular communication, and when bound to a ligand, Notch can release its intracellular segment and affect the transcription of the nucleus. Notch-induced transcription factor Sox9 promotes Sox2 transcription and enhances NOTCH1 expression in GSCs by upregulating Sox2 to attenuate the methylation of the NOTCH1 promoter. This positive feedback loop was associated with poor prognosis in a group of glioma subjects. These findings provide evidence that the NOTCH1-Sox2 positive feedback loop controls the invasion of GSCs along the white matter bundle.

Wnt signaling pathway: Recent studies have shown that Wnt/β-catenin can regulate MGMT gene expression in tumors and that inhibition of this gene expression can reduce drug resistance in tumor cells, which also provides a new therapeutic option for glioma chemotherapy. In malignant gliomas, Wnt inhibitory factor 1 (WIF1) expression impairs the stroma-dependent and stroma-non-dependent proliferation of tumor cells. Furthermore, overexpression of WIF1 induces a dose-dependent production of similarly sensitive cells in malignant tumor cells, and downregulation of WIF1 reveals an abnormal Wnt signaling pathway in 75% of glioma cells. Therefore, WIF1 expression may transform tumor cells into sensitive phenotypes for therapeutic purposes.

TGF-β signaling pathway: TGF-β is a vital cellular factor that regulates cell proliferation and differentiation through downstream Smad family signaling. Studies have shown that TGF-β can maintain the self-renewal property of GSCs through Sox2/4, while downregulating Sox2 can reduce the tumorigenicity of GSCs. TGF-β activation of Smad2/3/4 promotes LIF transcription, activating the JAK/STAT3 signaling pathway and enhancing stem cells' proliferation ability. In addition, TGF-β induces the expression of DNA-binding protein inhibitor 1 (ID1) in GSCs, which also promotes malignant cell proliferation of cells. The bone morphogenetic proteins (BMPs), named for their essential role in bone and cartilage formation, act by binding to kinase receptors on the cell surface and are also part of the TGF-β signaling pathway. BMPs regulate NSC proliferation and apoptosis and promote their differentiation. BMP ligands can reduce the number of tumor stem cells by inducing their differentiation into astrocytes. In vivo experiments with BMP treatment of tumor stem cells significantly delayed tumor growth and infiltration. Lee et al. reported differentiation of GSCs after BMP treatment, suggesting that selective activation of the BMP pathway may reduce the tumorigenic properties of GSCs.

RTK: The RTK family mediates multiple oncogenic growth factor pathways, with EGFR being the most prominent in gliomas. Malignant glioma cells frequently overexpress EGFR or express the variant EGFRvIII, which increases EGFR signaling. EGFRvIII transfection of mouse Nestin-positive neural stem cells induces glioma-like lesions, suggesting an important role for the EGFR signaling in glioma. In cell culture, the proliferation and neurosphere formation of GSCs is also dependent on EGFR, and signals elicited by RTK are transduced and amplified by downstream molecular cascades, such as the pro-survival AKT pathway. Once activated by RTK, AKT promotes tumor survival, proliferation, invasion, and secretion of pro-angiogenic factors. Pharmacological inhibitors of AKT can attenuate neurosphere formation, induce apoptosis, and even reduce intracranial tumor formation in GSCs, which have recently been shown to be more dependent on AKT signaling than other glioma cells. These data suggest that inhibition of AKT can specifically act on GSCs, thereby reducing the malignancy of gliomas. Other inhibitors of the MAPK pathway and mTOR pathway have also been tried for anti-glioma therapy.

4.3.2 Intracellular Signaling

Once the signaling pathway is activated, the cascade needs to be further extended from the cytoplasm to the nucleus to initiate the transcription of target genes. Transcription factors play a key role in this process, while miRNAs play a regulatory role. They act synergistically to influence the survival and proliferation of GSCs. Spanish scholars have sequenced the transcriptome of GSCs and found that transcription factors such as POU3F2, Sox2, SALL2, and Olig2 play a decisive role in the maintenance and regulation of GSCs. In collaboration with the UCSD group at the University of California, San Diego, our group found that c-Myc is critical in maintaining GSCs.

c-Myc: The critical role of c-Myc in normal stem cell and tumor cell growth has been extensively studied. c-Myc expression correlates with glioma grade and has recently been found to be upregulated in GSCs, and c-Myc is critical for both the survival of GSCs in vitro and tumorigenesis in vivo, a notion supported by murine glioma models. Murine astrocytes conditionally overexpressing c-Myc can lead to tumorigenesis, and in Tp53/Pten knockout mice, c-Myc can inhibit differentiation and promote self-renewal of tumor neurospheres. In collaboration with Prof. Clark Chen of UCSD, our group found that c-Myc knockdown significantly reduced the tumorigenic capacity of GBM cell lines. In contrast, overexpression of c-Myc resulted in significantly higher tumorigenic capacity in nude mice and higher expression of c-Myc in A2B5 positive cells. c-Myc expression is also epigenetically regulated, and LSD1 (lysine demethylase 1) can alter the expression of c-Myc. LSD1 can alter the methylation status of histone H3K4me3, and an increase in LSD1 can affect H3K4me3 and downregulate c-Myc expression, thus affecting the tumorigenicity of GSCs.

Octomer 4 (Oct4): Oct4, like Sox2 and Nanog, is an important factor in balancing the proliferation and differentiation of embryonic stem cells. Oct4 is highly expressed in many cell lines and human glioma specimens correlating with tumor grade. Additionally, Oct4 has been shown to interact with other transcription factors, such as Sox2, to maintain pluripotency and self-renewal in embryonic stem cells. A similar mechanism may be at work in GSCs. Although its direct role is unknown, overexpression of Oct4 in murine C6 glioma cells upregulates Nestin, suggesting that Oct4 may inhibit the differentiation of GSCs.

Olig2: Olig2 is a class of transcription factors that are almost exclusively expressed in the central nervous system. During brain development, Olig2 is expressed in neural progenitor cells that differentiate into oligodendrocytes and certain neuronal subtypes. Pathological analysis indicates that Olig2 is expressed in almost all adult astrocytomas and can induce tumors, suggesting an association with GSCs. From a functional perspective, Olig2 is required for normal NSCs and GSCs, and Olig2 maintains the replicative capacity of neural progenitor cells to ensure their multidirectional differentiation potential. In addition, Olig2 may regulate the proliferation of GSCs by inhibiting p21, a cell cycle regulator that controls the progression from the G1 phase to the S phase of the cell cycle. Olig2 is also involved in the regulation of various downstream target genes that play a critical role in the maintenance and proliferation of GSCs, such as PDGFRA, a receptor tyrosine kinase that is overexpressed in gliomas and plays a role in GSC proliferation and self-renewal.

BMI1: BMI1 belongs to the Polycomb group of genes and often functions as an upstream silencing gene. BMI1 has been found to determine the fate of many stem cells and has a positive effect on NSC self-renewal and is overexpressed in many tumors. In gliomas, BMI1 is overexpressed, and it is thought to be involved in the maintenance and progression of GSCs. Research has shown that BMI1 is required for the transformation of mature astrocytes and NSCs into HGGs in vivo. By comparing cells from wild-type and BMI1 knockout mice, researchers have demonstrated that BMI1 is equally important for transforming these two cell types. Furthermore, transformed wild-type NSCs induced HGG in vivo, while BMI1-deficient NSCs induced only some LGG, and very few of them expressed Nestin, suggesting a low number of GSCs. Although it is not clear whether BMI1 is equally important for human GSCs, the role of BMI1 in the maintenance of hepatocellular carcinoma stem cells has been confirmed.

miRNAs: miRNAs are small noncoding RNA molecules that regulate gene expression at the post-transcriptional level. In gliomas, dysregulation of miRNAs has been observed, and several miRNAs have been found to play important roles in the development and progression of gliomas, including GSCs. Some miRNAs, such as miRNA-21, are significantly overexpressed in GBM and can promote tumor growth and survival, while others, such as miRNA-145, are downregulated in HGGs and may have tumor suppressive roles. Overexpression of certain miRNAs, such as miRNA-21 and miRNA-145, can induce the differentiation of GSCs and reduce their proliferation. In addition, miRNA-451 is expressed at lower levels in GSCs compared to non-stem glioma cells and can inhibit the growth of GSCs and interfere with tumorsphere formation. Other miRNAs, such as miRNA-34a and miRNA-128, have also been implicated in regulating GSC proliferation and differentiation.

4.3.3 Cellular Signal Feedback to the Microenvironment

The interaction between tumor stem cells and their microenvironment is reciprocal, as tumor stem cells receive signals from extracellular sources through receptors and send signals to influence the microenvironment. Angiogenesis is the best example.

Active angiogenesis is an important hallmark of solid tumors, providing oxygen and nutrition to the tumor and even aiding in metastasis. Malignant gliomas are often rich in blood vessels, and the high number of neovascularization also suggests a high degree of malignancy and a poor clinical prognosis. GSCs play a crucial role in promoting angiogenesis, which is the formation of new blood vessels from pre-existing ones.

GSCs secrete various pro-angiogenic factors, such as VEGF, platelet-derived growth factor (PDGF), and basic fibroblast growth factor (bFGF), which stimulate the proliferation and migration of endothelial cells, the building blocks of blood vessels. In vitro and in vivo experiments have demonstrated that treatment of GSCs with the VEGF antibody bevacizumab attenuates their pro-angiogenic effect and has been permitted for use in glioma patients. The mechanism of VEGF is unclear, but hypoxia, acidosis, and oncogene activation may play a role. GSCs can also directly interact with endothelial cells through cell–cell contact and paracrine signaling, promoting their survival and sprouting.

In addition, GSCs can modify the extracellular matrix (ECM) surrounding blood vessels, making it more permissive for endothelial cell migration and invasion. GSCs can secrete enzymes such as matrix metalloproteinases (MMPs) that degrade the ECM, allowing endothelial cells to penetrate the surrounding tissues and form new blood vessels.

Furthermore, GSCs have been shown to promote the recruitment of pericytes, which are cells that provide structural support to blood vessels. Pericytes stabilize blood vessels and promote their maturation, thus improving their function. Furthermore, GSCs secrete factors such as PDGF and TGF-β that attract pericytes to blood vessels, which can enhance their survival and function. In addition, the stem cell nests mentioned above also reflect the interaction between GSCs and the microenvironment, and the relationship between GSCs and the microenvironment can also be found in the section "Glioma Stem Cells Are Involved in the Construction of the Glioma-Specific Microenvironment."

4.4 Treatment Targeting Glioma Stem Cells

GSCs are believed to be responsible for glioma initiation, progression, and resistance to current therapies. Thus, targeting GSCs has become an attractive therapeutic strategy for glioma treatment. Different approaches have been tested to target GSCs, including using small molecule inhibitors, monoclonal antibodies, and other agents. Currently, targeted therapies involving GSCs are divided into the following areas: modulation of signaling pathways, promotion of differentiation, enhancement of sensitivity to radiotherapy, indirect effects of stem cell nests, lytic virus therapy, and inhibition of adhesion molecules. The specific approaches are shown in Table 4.1.

Gene therapy has emerged as a promising approach for treating glioblastoma, as the occurrence and development of this aggressive brain tumor involve the regulation of many genes. The genetic modification of GSCs can affect their biological behaviors, such as proliferation and apoptosis. One commonly used gene therapy approach is thymidine kinase (TK)/ganciclovir (GCV) autocidal gene therapy. In this approach, the TK gene from herpes simplex virus type I is inserted into a suitable viral vector and delivered to GSCs. TK converts the antiviral drug GCV

Table 4.1 Targeted therapies for GSCs

Treatment principle	Target	Approach
Regulating signaling pathways	Notch	Gamma-secretase inhibitor
	PI3K pathway	AKT inhibitor
	Shh	Cyclopamine
	NF-kappaB pathway	The shRNA against A20
	c-Myc	shRNA against EZH2 or DANep
		Anti-c-Myc shRNA
	CXCR4	AMD 3100
	IL6	shRNA or antibody
Inhibitors of DNA repair pathways	PARPi	PARP inhibitor
Targeting GSCs specific markers	CD133, CD44 antibodies	Monoclonal antibodies

into a toxic metabolite, which induces stem cell death or apoptosis by blocking DNA synthesis through inhibition of DNA polymerase activity and misinsertion into the replicating DNA strand.

The viral vector with the suicide gene can be amplified in expression vector cells (VPC). By injecting VPCs into the brain and releasing the vector, the virus is highly selective in infecting tumor stem cells and does not damage the surrounding normal tissue. The TK gene product transferred to the nucleus accumulates in the cytoplasm. After injection of the nucleoside analog GCV, it is converted to the virulent ganocyclic guanosine triphosphate by TK. Guanosine triphosphate induces stem cell death or apoptosis by blocking DNA synthesis by inhibiting DNA polymerase activity and misinsertion into the replicating DNA strand.

Drugs targeting tumor stem cells are more effective in treating tumors, but current antitumor drugs are screened using tumor cell lines and have little effect on tumor stem cells. GSCs are one of the first solid tumor stem cells isolated and identified, and one of the very few tumor stem cells that can be cultured in vitro for a long period, which is an important model in tumor stem cell research. In addition to forming neurosphere-like clusters in suspension culture, GSCs can also be cultured for long periods of time in adherent culture conditions which is highly beneficial for high-throughput screening. Unlike primary glioblastoma cell culture in a serum-containing medium, the genome and gene expression profile of GSCs are extremely stable under long-term culture conditions. Therefore, GSCs are ideal for screening antitumor stem cell drugs.

The discovery and study of GSCs have undoubtedly advanced our understanding of glioma, but there are still many issues in this area that need further investigation, which can be broadly listed as follows. First, we need to find more specific markers for GSCs. Although CD133 is currently the most commonly used marker for GSCs, it has been found that CD133-negative cells may also be stem cells. Therefore more specific markers would not only help us to define GSCs but also provide more accurate targets for targeted therapy. Secondly, to clarify the origin of GSCs, the relationship between GSCs and normal adult NSCs and progenitor cells is not clear, and if we can understand what kind of cells are generated by the mutation of GSCs during the progression of glioma, we can establish a new classification of glioma based on GSCs, which may better indicate the prognosis and even guide the treatment. Then, the escape of GSCs from conventional therapies has always been a problem, and further insight into the signal transduction mechanisms involved will be a key aspect of GSCs research. Finally, the development and improvement of targeted therapies. However, since GSCs share many genes and antigens with normal adult NSCs and progenitor cells, precisely targeting and avoiding damaging normal cells is an important issue to consider in these emerging therapies.

Further Reading

Brescia P, Ortensi B, Fornasari L, et al. CD133 is essential for glioblastoma stem cell maintenance. Stem Cells. 2013;31(5):857–69.

Campos B, Gal Z, Baader A, et al. Aberrant self-renewal and quiescence contribute to the aggressiveness of glioblastoma. J Pathol. 2014;234(1):23–33.

Cheng L, Huang Z, Zhou W, et al. Glioblastoma stem cells generate vascular pericytes to support vessel function and tumor growth. Cell. 2013;153(1):139–52.

Ciceroni C, Bonelli M, Mastrantoni E, et al. Type-3 metabotropic glutamate receptors regulate chemo-resistance in glioma stem cells, and their levels are inversely related to survival in patients with malignant gliomas. Cell Death Differ. 2013;20(3):396–407.

Jackson M, Hassiotou F, Nowak A, et al. Glioblastoma stem-like cells: at the root of tumor recurrence and a therapeutic target. Carcinogenesis. 2015;36(2):177–85.

Jun HJ, Bronson RT, Charest A. Inhibition of EGFR induces a c-MET-driven stem cell population in glioblastoma. Stem Cells. 2014;32(10):338–48.

Kozono D, Li J, Nitta M, et al. Dynamic epigenetic regulation of glioblastoma tumorigenicity through LSD1 modulation of MYC expression. Proc Natl Acad Sci USA. 2015;112(30):E4055–64.

Lan X, Jörgd J, Cavallif MG, et al. Fate mapping of human glioblastoma reveals an invariant stem cell hierarchy. Nature. 2017;549(7671):227–32.

Nakano I. Stem cell signature in glioblastoma: therapeutic development for a moving target. J Neurosurg. 2015;122(2):324–30.

Wang R, Chadalavada K, Wilshire J, et al. Glioblastoma stem-like cells give rise to tumour endothelium. Nature. 2010;468(7325):829–33.

Wei H, Yao Y, Liangfu Z. Advances in the study of tumor stem cell markers in malignant glioma. Chin J Surg. 2011a;49(10):944–6.

Wei H, Yao Y, Yiwei C, et al. Phase I clinical trial of human glioma stem cell-like antigen-sensitized dendritic cell vaccine. Chin J Neurosurg. 2011b;27(1):90–3.

5 Advances in Tumor Microenvironment of Gliomas

Wei Hua, Hui Yang, and Qi Yue

In 1978, Schofield proposed the "microenvironment" hypothesis to describe the physiological microenvironment that supports stem cell growth. The tumor microenvironment, which is the internal environment in which tumor cells arise and live, includes not only the tumor cells themselves but also the surrounding fibroblasts, immune and inflammatory cells, glial cells, as well as the matrix, microvasculature, and cellular molecules that infiltrate the extracellular area. Due to its unique proliferation and development processes, a tumor disrupts the normal internal environment and creates a favorable tissue environment for its growth. This leads to the formation of a tumor microenvironment that is markedly different from the normal tissue environment, featuring characteristics such as hypoxia, acidosis, interstitial hypertension, high levels of growth factors, immune-inflammatory reactions, and protein hydrolases, among others.

The special microenvironment leads to unique characteristics of tumors, such as resistance to apoptosis, genomic instability, signals for sustained proliferation, evasion of growth inhibition, immune escape, aberrant angiogenesis, invasion, and migration. These characteristics lead to the unsatisfactory effect of conventional treatments such as surgical resection, radiotherapy, and chemotherapy. They also result in tumor metastasis and recurrence, as well as poor prognosis for patients.

W. Hua · H. Yang · Q. Yue (✉)
Department of Neurosurgery, Huashan Hospital, Fudan University, Shanghai, China

5.1 Glioma Stem Cells Are Involved in the Construction of the Glioma-Specific Microenvironment

GSCs are the root cause of glioma occurrence and development. They exist in a specific microenvironment known as the stem cell niche, which provides similar circumstances for GSC as the normal stem cells live in. Specifically, the stem cell niche helps GSC maintain undifferentiated and self-renewing by producing signals and growth factors that contribute to the maintenance of stemness. GSCs intrinsically regulate core molecular pathways, such as c-Myc, Oct4, Olig2, and BMI1, which may be involved in the BMI1/TP53/Rb signaling pathway, TGF-β signaling pathway, Wnt signaling pathway, Notch signaling pathway, and Hedgehog/Nanog signaling pathway. GSCs are also influenced by interactions with the intercellular and extracellular matrix.

Recent studies have shown that the interaction between GSCs and the microenvironment is bidirectional, and this bidirectional interaction may affect the fate of tumor cells. This section will briefly review the research on the relationship

Y. Mao (ed.), *Progress in the Diagnosis and Treatment of Gliomas*, Experts' Perspectives on Medical Advances, https://doi.org/10.1007/978-981-99-0123-4_5

between GSCs and the vascular microenvironment, hypoxic microenvironment, and immune microenvironment. For further information, please refer to the sections on "Advances in Glioma Stem Cell Research" and "Immunotherapy and Oncolytic Virus Would Provide New Adjuvant Therapy."

Studies have shown that the vascular microenvironment can make GSCs tolerant to chemotherapy and radiotherapy by activating the AKT/PKB signaling pathway. GSCs are located around the vascular microenvironment, and disruption of the vascular microenvironment can destroy GSCs. GSCs can also promote angiogenesis by secreting VEGF, etc. Solid tumors can form intratumorally hypoxic areas due to their high proliferation rate. Studies have shown that GSCs are more tolerant to hypoxia than differentiated cells, and the hypoxic microenvironment plays a critical role in maintaining the survival of GSCs. Hypoxia can promote GSCs proliferation, which may be directly related to HIF-1α and HIF-2α. The researchers examined the hypoxic response of GSCs and confirmed that the hypoxia-inducible factor HIF-2α and multiple HIF-regulated genes are preferentially expressed in GSCs compared to bulk tumor cells and normal neural precursor cells. Targeting HIFs in GSCs inhibits their self-renewal, proliferation, and survival and diminishes the tumorigenic capacity of GSCs in vivo.

Despite systematic immune surveillance in an organism, GSCs can evade immune surveillance by altering surface antigens, expressing immune escape-related molecules, and inducing immunosuppressive cells and cytokines. In addition, interstitial cells in their microenvironment are also involved.

5.2 Tumor Microenvironment and Blood Vessels

5.2.1 Angiogenesis-Related Cells

Gliomas are typically well-supplied with blood, and mounting evidence suggests that the glioma vascular system, comprising of endothelial cells, perivascular cells, and astrocytes, plays a role in tumor progression. The concept of the perivascular niche (PVN) has emerged, underscoring the importance of the blood supply system in the glioma microenvironment. HGG is characterized by endothelial cell hyperplasia and microvascular hyperplasia, which involve overgrowth of endothelial cells, perivascular cells, and vascular smooth muscle cells that make up the microvasculature. This area of angiogenesis represents the site of tumor progression and invasion.

PVN is a crucial site for the aggregation of brain tumor stem cells. In normal brain tissue, NSCs are predominantly found in the perivascular region, facilitating their maintenance and interaction with endothelial and other stromal cells. Similarly, in the PVN region of glioma tissue, glioma stem cells (GSCs) interact with endothelial and stromal cells in their microenvironment to maintain stemness. In vitro experiments have shown that GSCs co-cultured with endothelial cells are more tightly bound than normal neurons and exhibit better self-renewal ability, indicating that direct cell contact-mediated signaling in PVN may be critical for tumor progression. PVN can also recruit bone marrow-derived cells during development, including endothelial progenitor cells, perivascular primitive cells, and CD45+ cells. Endothelial progenitor cells differentiate into vascular endothelial cells, while perivascular primitive cells develop into perivascular and smooth muscle cells, which form the vascular system. In addition, some $CD45^{+}$ cells differentiate into perivascular macrophages and microglia.

In normal brain tissue, the vasculature is surrounded by perivascular cells and vascular smooth muscle cells, which play a crucial role in maintaining vascular morphology and hemodynamic stability. They do this by recruiting perivascular cells and smooth muscle cells to PDGFB-expressing endothelial cells. In the tumor microenvironment, the recruitment of perivascular and smooth muscle cells is important for maintaining the stability of PVN morphology and the activity of tumor endothelial cells. It has been shown that this recruitment promotes microvascular hyperproliferation, while NG2 expressed by perivascular cells has been shown to promote glioma cell proliferation. Other studies have also shown that perivascular cell recruitment promotes angiogenesis in tumor tissues, and HIF-1α may be involved in perivascular cell aggregation in PVN.

Vascular endothelial cells play a crucial role in tumor progression. In addition to their long-recognized function as suppliers of nutrients and oxygen to tumor cells, they also sustain tumor stem cell activity by providing relevant cytokines and promoting intra-tumor angiogenesis. Time-lapse microscopy of rat glioma sections demonstrated that Nestin- and CD133-positive GSCs were inserted between closely packed vascular endothelium during migration. The number of GSCs arranged along the vessel wall was positively correlated with tumor grade. Additionally, vascular endothelial cells secrete nitric oxide (NO) that enhances the self-renewal and tumorigenic capacity of GSCs, and inhibiting NO synthesis by NO synthase inhibitors can prolong the survival of tumor-bearing mice.

VEGF, a growth factor that acts directly on vascular endothelial cells, has been shown to regulate endothelial cell proliferation, promote angiogenesis, and participate in the regulation of tumor proliferation. The specific binding of VEGF to its receptor VEGFR2 activates vascular endothelial cell proliferation and promotes angiogenesis, while regulating endothelial cell permeability. Moreover, neuropilin-1 (NRP1), a VEGF co-receptor, enhances the binding of VEGF to VEGFR2, and its expression is closely related to the clinicopathological characteristics and prognosis of glioma.

5.2.2 Glioma Vasculogenic Mimicry and the Tumor Microenvironment

Vasculogenic mimicry (VM) is a unique luminal structure formed by interconnected tumor cells without endothelial cell coverage, first identified by Maniotis et al. in uveal malignant melanoma. This special structure plays a crucial role in constructing the tumor microenvironment and provides structural support for tumor development. Tissue sections stained for VMs reveal that they are lined with tumor cells, with a large number of laminins surrounding the tumor cells to form spherical nests. Unlike the traditional concept of angiogenesis, light microscopy, transmission electron microscopy, and immunohistochemistry did not detect any endothelial cells in the lumen surrounded by a large amount of stroma.

In glioma, VM was identified in a glioma model in nude mice, and the lumen that was CD34-negative and PAS-positive was VM, while the lumen that was double positive for CD34 and PAS was endothelial vascular, and both lumens showed erythrocytes but no necrosis. The presence of VM structures was associated with poor prognosis, and in VM-positive aggressive tumors, vascular wall cell-related genes such as tissue factor (TF), tissue factor pathway (TFP) inhibitor, and endothelial vasculature were found to be involved in the glioma microenvironment.

VM-positive aggressive tumors exhibit endothelial-like anticoagulation mechanisms, and the tubular meshwork contains both plasma and blood cells, implying that the endothelium-free meshwork formed by the arrangement of tumor cells can facilitate blood flow in vivo. VM is the main mode of blood supply in the early stage of tumor growth. As the tumor grows, endothelial cells differentiate and proliferate to form mosaic-like vessels as a transitional mode. Finally, endothelium-dependent vessels replace VM and mosaic-like vessels as the main mode of blood supply in the later stage of tumor growth. Therefore, VM may be the main source of blood supply to tumor tissues in the early stages when endothelium-dependent vessels are unable to cope with malignant tumor growth due to the need for outgrowth and recruitment of endothelial cells.

Regulators of VM formation are currently the focus of research, but the exact mechanisms are not well understood. Some studies have found that a large number of cells increased their expression of VEGF, the cyclooxygenase during VM formation, while matrix metalloproteinases, pathway inhibitors of the tissue factor pathway, involve the regulation of VM formation. In gliomas, CD133+ tumor cells are more likely to form VMs, and studies have suggested that VM wall cells have the same phenotype as GSCs. Evidence for the transdifferentiation of GSCs into endothelial cells has also been provided, including the slab-like morphology of GSCs in endothelial cytokine-inducible medium, which has an ultrastructure similar to that of vascular endothelial cells. Additionally, GSCs can transdifferentiate into vascular smooth muscle-like cells expressing the vascular wall markers SMA and PDGFRβ, suggesting that they may be able to differentiate into vascular endothelial progenitor cells or mature endothelial cells.

Factors that both promote and inhibit angiogenesis can affect the internal vascular architecture of a tumor through autocrine, endocrine, and paracrine forms involving various cytokines secreted directly or through exosomes. In one study, exosomes from the blood and cerebrospinal fluid of GBM patients were extracted and applied to endothelial cells, which were found to be abnormally activated by AKT/β-catenin and subsequently exhibited altered proliferation and invasive capacity. Previous studies based on microfluidic technology have found that U87 glioma cell line-derived exosomes containing DLL4, an important ligand of the Notch signaling pathway, could increase endothelial cell motility, and this new means of intercellular communication provides a promising model for anti-vascular therapy in the future.

5.3 Glioma Microenvironment and Glioma Invasion

Gliomas, especially GBM, are highly aggressive tumors that do not have a clear border with normal brain tissue, which is one of the reasons why they are so difficult to cure.

The glioma invasion mainly involves three processes: (1) adhesion of tumor cells to ECM; (2) degradation of ECM; and (3) migration and angiogenesis of tumor cells. In these processes, the tumor microenvironment plays a regulatory role in the invasion of tumors.

The main factors associated with ECM degradation are MMPs, urokinase-type plasminogen activator (uPA), and proteases (cathepsins), among others. MMPs are particularly effective in degrading almost all protein components of the ECM. Studies have shown that the expression of MMP-2 and MMP-9 is significantly increased in human glioma tissues, and their levels correlate positively with tumor malignancy. uPA and uPA receptors can directly degrade the ECM and basement membrane by activating fibrinogen into fibrinolytic enzymes. Both in vivo and in vitro experiments have demonstrated that downregulation of MMP-9, uPA receptor, and cathepsin B expression can inhibit the activation of integrin signaling, thus reducing the invasive ability of gliomas.

Non-tumor cells in the glioma microenvironment are involved in regulating the tumor invasion process. Fibroblasts in gliomas can promote tumor angiogenesis and metastasis by activating tumor cells. Co-culture of brain-derived primary fibroblasts and primary glioma cells upregulates tumor invasion by promoting the activity of MMP-2 and its activators, MT1-MMP and MT2-MMP, in tumor cells. Co-culture of astrocytes with CD133+ GSCs also significantly upregulates the invasive ability of GSCs. Additionally, tumor-associated macrophages (TAMs), fibroblasts, and some lymphocytes secrete cytokines and chemokines that regulate the aggressive behavior of tumors, leading to the upregulation of the invasive ability of GSCs. Cell adhesion molecules, including the integrin family, selectin family, and immunoglobulin superfamily, are also involved in cell-to-cell and cell-to-ECM adhesion.

EGFR and EGFRvIII can activate MMP-1, MMP-13, and fibroblast activation protein (FAP), enhancing the invasive ability of GBM. The expression of wild-type EGFR in human GBM specimens was positively correlated with the degree of GBM invasion; studies in mouse glioma models have shown that the ability of EGFRvIII to promote tumor cell invasion was correlated with the activation of STAT3 and the activation of MMP-1 and MMP-13, etc. VEGF is closely related to tumor angiogenesis, and early studies have suggested that VEGF significantly promotes glioma angiogenesis. However, recent studies have shown that VEGF inhibits glioma invasion by recruiting protein tyrosine phosphatase 1B (PTP1B), suggesting that VEGF may play a two-way regulatory role on glioma invasion.

Several enzymes in the glioma microenvironment also influence the invasive process of glioma. The glioma team at the Department of Neurosurgery, Huashan Hospital, Fudan University, found that the expression level of Capn4, a member of the calpain family, was positively correlated with tumor grade. Knockdown of Capn4 expression by RNA interference revealed that Capn4-high-expressing gliomas exhibited more aggression and implied a poorer prognosis. Further studies showed that Capn4 regulates miR-124 expression and affects MMP-2 levels, thereby influencing the aggressiveness of gliomas.

5.4 The Immune Microenvironment of Glioma Is Unique

5.4.1 The Concept of Immune Privilege in the CNS Has Undergone a Shift in Recent Decades

The blood–brain barrier (BBB) is no longer viewed as a static barrier that completely prevents the exchange of cells and molecules but rather as a regulatory system that controls the exchange of substances between the CNS and the periphery. During inflammation, immune lymphocytes can migrate into the CNS in response to cytokines such as IFN-γ and IFN-α and β-integrins, as well as matrix metalloproteins. Soluble immune-related factors, like immunoglobulins, can also cross the BBB via carrier-mediated transport by FcRn, an immunoglobulin receptor expressed in various tissues.

The conventional wisdom that the CNS lacks a traditional lymphatic system, contains few antigen-presenting cells (APCs), and has a weak immune response to foreign antigens led to the notion that the brain is an "immune privilege" tissue. However, as research progresses, there is growing evidence that the CNS contains a robust innate and adaptive immune system that responds dynamically to different contexts. Furthermore, the CNS possesses components that regulate the immunomodulatory properties of local immune responses, which could be present in other organs of the body. Thus, the traditional concept of CNS immune privilege is outdated, and it is more accurate to view the CNS as a dynamic system that can adapt to its environment.

The traditional belief that the CNS is immune privileged due to the absence of a lymphatic system has been disproven. Soluble antigens from the CNS can enter peripheral lymph nodes, and tracer studies have shown that CNS antigens can reach the nasal mucosa via the CSF pathway. Under homeostatic conditions, dendritic cells in peripheral lymph nodes capture CNS-derived antigens in a similar manner to antigens produced elsewhere in the body. However, the CNS is relatively deficient in immune cells, especially in the brain parenchyma, which is maintained in a resting state by the blood–brain barrier endothelium. The CSF-draining spaces, on the other hand, contain antigen-presenting cells that respond to foreign antigens in the same way as other organs.

The barrier that prevents leukocyte from entering into the brain parenchyma consists of the CSF-draining Virchow–Robin perivascular gap located posterior to the endothelium and the glial boundary membrane, which is the astrocyte peduncle barrier between the perivascular gap and the brain parenchyma. In addition to forming a second mechanical barrier to immune cells, the Virchow–Robin gap is a very important component of the inflammatory response, as the astrocyte peduncle expresses the death ligand FasL/CD95L, which induces apoptosis of T cells by binding with the Fas receptor on the surface of T cells and suppresses the inflammatory response.

Thus, most inflammatory cells that enter the Virchow–Robin gap at homeostasis are retained in the perivascular space and do not continue to cross the glial boundary membrane. In the disease state, the integrity of the blood–brain barrier is disrupted, and large numbers of circulating immune cells infiltrate the brain parenchyma. For more detailed information about antigen presentation in the CNS and peripheral tissues can be found in the following section on "Antigen Presentation in the Glioma Microenvironment."

Although the exact mechanisms by which the central nervous system coordinates immune responses are not yet fully understood, there is mounting evidence that some of the immunoregulatory processes observed in the brain can also be observed in other tissues throughout the body. For instance, the FasL is expressed not only in astrocytes but also in various peripheral tissues including lymphoid tissue, liver, testis, and transverse muscle. In the testis, there is a blood–tissue barrier formed by tight intercellular junctions similar to that of the central nervous system.

In addition, several organs, including the brain, liver, and gastrointestinal tract, secrete immunomodulatory factors that enhance the expression of Treg and induce local immune tolerance. Therefore, as therapeutic approaches to overcome the blood–brain barrier immunomodulatory mechanism are making progression, they may also bring benefits to immunotherapy in other similar organs.

5.4.2 Antigen Presentation in the Glioma Microenvironment

Typically, exogenous antigens are captured and phagocytosed at the cell surface before being presented to CD4+ T lymphocytes via binding to specific APC surface MHC class II molecules. Meanwhile, endogenous antigens are processed by the intracellular rough endoplasmic reticulum and then bound to APC surface MHC class I molecules for presentation to CD8+ T lymphocytes. However, the expression of tumor antigens involves a third approach known as "cross-presentation": tumor antigens generated by dead tumor cell lysis bind to MHC class I molecules and are further presented to CD8+ T lymphocytes, thereby triggering an adaptive immune response against the tumor cells.

Although the presence of antigen-presenting cells has been demonstrated in the central nervous system, the question of whether CNS tumor antigen presentation begins in the brain or in the periphery remains inconclusive. Given the existence of the blood–brain barrier, microglia are generally considered to be the main antigen-presenting cells in the brain. Both in vivo and in vitro experiments have demonstrated the ability of microglia to cross-present antigens. Systemic irradiation could deplete intracranial and peripheral dendritic cells and macrophages. Jarry et al. established a murine irradiation model with intracranial OVA antigen injection. CD8 T-cell activation was found to be weaker in the irradiation-treated group than in the control group, which also confirmed the antigen-presenting properties of intracranial dendritic cells. The tumor-infiltrating dendritic cells may also play an important role in glioma antigen presentation, and their ability to present antigens may be stronger than that of microglia.

However, the ability of microglia and tumor-infiltrating dendritic cells to activate CD8+ T cells in the glioma microenvironment remains unknown. Research has shown that high concentrations of immunosuppressive cytokines, such as TGF-β, IL-10, and PGE2, downregulate the expression of MHC molecules on the surface of microglia in the glioma microenvironment. Even when isolated from glioma tissue and stimulated, microglia exhibit lower MHC expression than normal microglia. Microglia in the glioma microenvironment also secrete 50% more TNF-α and exhibit higher levels of STAT3 activation and IL-10 secretion. Additionally, IL-10 inhibits dendritic cell maturation and maintains dormant dendritic cells. These results suggest that antigen-presenting cells adopt an immunosuppressive phenotype with suppressed antigen-presenting ability in the glioma microenvironment.

In addition to microglia and dendritic cells, TAMs, B cells, and perivascular cells are important for tumor antigen presentation in the CNS. TAMs are even more abundant in glioma tissues than microglia and, as confirmed in a mouse model of multiple sclerosis, are believed to be more important for antigen presentation. However, there is no accepted method for distinguishing between these two cell phenotypes, making it impossible to precisely compare the antigen-presenting capacity of microglia and macrophages.

Conventionally, T-cell immunity has been considered the key component of antitumor immunity. However, recent studies have revealed that B cells also have antigen-presenting capacity and contribute to antitumor immunity, a function that is increasingly being recognized in the central nervous system. For instance, adenovirus-mediated intravenous administration of herpes simplex virus type I TK and tyrosine kinase3 (Ad-Flt3L) can recruit antigen-presenting cells and kill tumor cells. This method prolongs the survival of 60% of wild-type mice but is ineffective in B-cell-deficient mice. The transcription factor BLIMP1 is essential for the terminal differentiation of B cells into antibody-secreting plasma cells. No significant survival difference was observed between Blimp-1-deficient mice and wild-type mice, suggesting that tumor suppressive efficacy of B cell is not related to the production of tumor-associated antibodies.

While perivascular cells have traditionally been thought to play a crucial role in regulating blood flow, vascular permeability, and vascular remodeling in arterioles, venules, and capillaries, recent studies have demonstrated that they also have phagocytic and antigen-presenting capabilities. In brain capillaries, perivascular cells are highly sensitive to inflammatory cytokines, and inflammatory factors such as TNF-α and IFN-γ are thought to increase their antigen-presenting abilities and elevate MHC class II antigen expression. Nevertheless, it is still unclear whether perivascular cells in the glioma microenvironment can cross-present antigens. The pathways by which the glioma microenvironment regulates their antigen presentation ability remain to be explored.

5.4.3 Immune Factors in the Glioma Microenvironment

Some cytokines have a wide range of biologically active effects that mediate tumor cell proliferation, invasion, and immune escape. Therefore, cytokine-specific therapies have very promising prospects for both systemic and intracranial tumors. However, a major challenge in cytokine therapy is the pleiotropic and biphasic immunomodulatory effects of these cytokines, as well as the adverse effects of the "cytokine storm."

IL-10: IL-10 is a classical immunosuppressive factor that is secreted by numerous cells of the innate and adaptive immune systems, such as antigen-presenting cells and CD4+ helper T cells, as well as by intracranial and systemic malignancies. IL-10 binds to IL-10 receptors on the surface of dendritic cells to activate STAT3 transcriptional regulators, which in turn promote the secretion of IL-6, TNF-α, and IL-1β, upregulate IL-10 secretion, and maintain the immature state of dendritic cells. In macrophages, monocytes and dendritic cells, IL-10 inhibits the ability of cells to present antigens by activating MARCH1. IL-10 also impedes the effects of cytotoxic T cells by inducing and maintaining the expression of the Tregs transcription factor Foxp3. Paradoxically, IL-10 can also exert pro-inflammatory and antitumor effects by effectively stimulating the activation of NK cells, mast cells, and B cells and by enhancing the cytotoxic activity of CD8+ T cells in concert with other cytokines. IL-10 could inhibit the promoter of angiogenic factors to suppress angiogenesis, and it has been shown to inhibit tumor growth in certain preclinical tumor models.

It has long been shown that in vivo glioma tissue can secrete IL-10, and the mRNA expression level of IL-10 is positively correlated with tumor grade in astrocytoma. However, glioma cells do not directly secrete IL-10 but produce soluble cytokines that induce IL-10 secretion by TAMs and microglia.

In addition, IL-10 displayed a dose-dependent manner enhancing glioma proliferation and invasion in in vitro studies. However, recent studies have also shown that vaccination with tumor-antigen-loaded dendritic cells can suppress tumor growth by stimulating glioma-associated T cells to secrete IL-10 continuously. This process, in which IL-10 may interact with IFN-γ, inhibits tumor growth by regulating indoleamine 2,3 dioxygenase (IDO)-mediated histidine metabolism in glioma-associated antigen-presenting cells. The tumor suppressive function of IDO will be discussed later.

In summary, IL-10 has a two-sided effect on glioma growth, closely related to the physiological microenvironment in which the tumor is located. While IL-10 from TAMs exhibits overall pro-tumor and immunosuppressive effects, high IL-10 concentrations sustained and secreted by T-cells also have immune-promoting and tumor-suppressive effects. During immunotherapy, we should recognize the specific microenvironment in which IL-10-secreting cells are located and effectively kill tumor-promoting IL-10-secreting cells.

TGF-β: TGF-β is a cytokine that has a molecular weight of 25 kDa that is secreted by various cell types such as immune cells and malignant tumor cells; it is highly pleiotropic and regulates a variety of biological functions such as cell proliferation, migration, angiogenesis, embryonic stem cell differentiation, and immune surveillance. The Smad complex regulates the expression of genes related to immunosuppression, angiogenesis, and cell proliferation in the nucleus. They also play diverse roles in tumorigenesis, inhibiting early tumor proliferation and promoting advanced tumor progression. TGF-β expression has been found to correlate with tumor grade and malignancy in many intracranial and systemic tumors, such as prostate, small cell lung, pancreatic, and gastric cancers. Early findings identified TGF-β2 as a key factor in the immunosuppression of glioma-associated T cells. Since then, researchers have been working to investigate the relevance of some of the factors involved in tumor immunosuppression to tumorigenesis. TGF-β was originally isolated from the sera of patients with malignant glioma and was appropriately described as a "humoral immunosuppressor"; soluble TGF-β significantly suppressed lymphocyte function and induced apoptosis of lymphocytes, especially CD4+ helper T cells. Subsequent studies over the next few decades have further elucidated that TGF-β reduces the cytotoxic effects of immune cells and promotes immune escape and glioma growth. TGF-β also promotes the conversion of T cells and monocytes to an immunosuppressive phenotype, which further promotes an immune-tolerant state and facilitates tumor growth. In addition, TGF-β can also promote glioma growth and metastasis by activating angiogenesis, thereby sustaining the generation of GSCs, inducing platelet-derived growth factors that act as autocrine proliferative signals for glioma cells, and promoting the synthesis of matrix metalloproteases.

TGF-β signaling blockade has been shown to rescue antitumor immune function in gliomas in preclinical models. In vitro experiments have shown that knockdown TGF-β in glioma cell lines increased their sensitivity to immune-promoting factors. In a mouse glioma model, the mice administrated with oral TGF-β1 receptor inhibitor sx-007 showed significantly longer survival. Also, the mice treated with sx-007 exhibited higher levels of CD8+ T cells in brain tissue compared to the control group, suggesting that TGF-β depletion reversed the immunosuppressive effect.

Both in vivo and in vitro studies have shown that radiotherapy induces high expression of TGF-β. Therefore, TGF-β-neutralizing antibodies may not only overcome TGF-β-induced tumor immune suppression but also improve the sensitivity of radiotherapy. In vitro experiments have demonstrated that the TGF-β R1 kinase inhibitor LY2109761 can improve the sensitivity of glioma cell lines and tumor stem cells to radiotherapy. Several TGF-β-targeted glioma therapeutics are already in clinical trials, the most promising of which is Trabedersen, an oligoclonal nucleotide antagonist of TGF-β2 mRNA, which has been proven to inhibit tumor proliferation and enhance antitumor immunity in vitro. Phase I/II clinical trials have demonstrated that Trabedersen prolongs survival in treatment-refractory HGG. The subsequent phase IIb RCT also demonstrated that Trabedersen significantly prolonged the 2-year survival of refractory anaplastic astrocytoma compared to conventional chemotherapy, but due to methodological flaws, these findings were not widely accepted. Phase I and II trials of LY2157299, another TGF-β receptor kinase inhibitor, in primary and recurrent GBM, have also concluded, and results will be available soon.

IDO: IDO is an intracellular enzyme secreted mainly by macrophages and dendritic cells and is mainly associated with inflammation-related factors such as IFN-γ, IFN-α, IFN-β, and lipopolysaccharide. IDO catalyzes the rate-limiting step of tryptophan metabolism and promotes the production of kynurenine, which has a suppressive effect on immune system function. At the same time, kynurenine can promote Treg cell proliferation and inhibit cytotoxic T cells' function. IDO is expressed in many intracranial or systemic tumors, such as glioma, lung, prostate, colon, and pancreatic cancers and is negatively associated with prognosis in tumor patients. This also proves the role of Treg in promoting tumor progression. Under normal physiological conditions, brain tissue does not contain IDO, while it is present in glioma tissue, and its expression is positively correlated with the degree of tumor malignancy. Its role in tumor progression is related to the recruitment of restrictive T cells, with CCL22 playing a crucial role. Recent studies have shown that gliomas mainly self-secrete IDO rather than it being secreted by tumor-associated macrophages, microglia, or dendritic cells, whereas, in other tumors, IDO is mainly secreted by dendritic cells. The intracranial xenograft model by GL261 cell line in wild-type and IDO-deficient mice showed no significant correlation between survival or intratumoral T-cell recruitment and IDO concentration. However, IDO-secreting GL261 tumor-bearing mice showed higher intratumoral Treg infiltration and shorter survival.

5.4.4 Lymphocyte Subpopulations in the Glioma Microenvironment Are Predominantly Immunosuppressive

Treg: Treg, a diverse subset of T helper cells, plays a critical role in promoting immunosuppression and immune tolerance. While these cells regulate autoimmunity, they can also impede antitumor immune responses and promote tumor growth. Malignant tumors actively recruit Treg populations, and studies have shown that Treg is associated with higher tumor grade and poorer prognosis in high-density tumors. Treg is believed to play a pivotal role in tumorigenesis and progression, and its immunosuppressive effect contributes to the failure of immunotherapy. In a previous study, we found that Treg infiltration in GBM was closely related to patient survival and could be used for prognosis prediction. The study included 62 GBM patients who underwent tumor resection between 2006 and 2010 in the Department of Neurosurgery, Huashan Hospital, Fudan University. Primary GBM specimens were subjected to IHC staining targeting Foxp3, CD8, TP53, MGMT, and Ki-67. Cases were classified based on the number of positive cells under the microscope, and clinical data were statistically analyzed. The results showed that GBM patients with a higher degree of Treg infiltration in the tumor tissues had shorter survival, suggesting that Treg is an independent prognostic factor for GBM and a promising target for immunotherapy in the future.

Treg accounts for 5–10% of total CD4+ T cells and can be classified into primary regulatory T cells of thymic origin (nTreg) and adaptive regulatory T cells of peripheral blood origin (iTreg). Based on the current evaluation methods, it is suggested that Treg infiltrated in malignant glioma is mainly nTreg rather than iTreg. In the murine glioma model, Treg infiltration in the tumor was significantly reduced in the mice with thymectomy before tumor formation compared with the mice in the control group. In addition, it was shown that more than 90% of the tumor Treg expresses Helios transcription factors, which was found primarily in nTreg rather than iTreg, reinforcing the idea that tumor-associated Treg mainly originated from thymus. Although the exact mechanism remains unclear, there is growing evidence that gliomas may secrete cytokines recruiting nTreg. Among them, CCL22 secreted by gliomas may play a major role by specifically binding to the lymphocyte surface ligand CCR4, which has been shown to be widely expressed in tumor-infiltrating Treg. In vitro experiments have also confirmed the chemotactic effect of CCL22 on Treg.

Conventional therapies targeting Treg are nonspecific and reduce their abundance by using anti-CD25 antibodies and cyclophosphamide. It is still unclear whether these methods target nTreg or iTreg. However, based on the consensus that infiltrating regulatory T cells in intracranial and systemic tumors are predominantly nTreg, it may be possible to devise targeted strategies for nTreg depletion that minimize adverse effects and limit systemic Treg depletion. For example, nTreg cells are thought to exert immunosuppressive effects primarily through cell contact-dependent mechanisms, including the coinhibitory molecules CTLA-4 and PD-L1, membrane-bound TGF-β, adenosine and granzyme B, perforin, and the Fas/FasL pathway. Thus, it may be possible to modulate nTreg activity by blocking the interaction between ligands and receptors on the surface of these immune cells. Another possible route for Treg-targeted therapy is to disrupt the CCL22-CCR4 pathway. Depletion of CCR4+ regulatory T cells with anti-CCR4 antibodies has recently been reported to preserve naive T cells in patients with melanoma.

Microglia and monocyte-derived macrophages: Microglia and monocyte-derived macrophages are the two major types of glioma-associated myeloid cells. Microglia are the resident immune cells of the central nervous system, accounting for 5–20% of all glial cells, and play an important role in the innate immune system of the brain. In contrast, monocyte-derived macrophages are generally restricted to perivascular, choroidal, and meningeal sites and enter the brain parenchyma only in disease states or when inflammation disrupts the integrity of the blood–brain barrier. In gliomas, monocyte-derived macrophages and microglia account for up to 30% of total tumor tissue cells. It has been reported that HGG tends to exhibit higher levels of monocyte-derived macrophage and microglia aggregation than LGG.

Recent work has progressively demonstrated that microglia and tumor-associated macrophages are distinct subpopulations developed from the mononuclear phagocyte system. However, it has been a challenge to distinguish between these two subpopulations in glioma tissues. In the past, the integrin CD11b and the leukocyte surface antigen CD45 have been used to distinguish between these two cell types—microglia with high CD11b expression and low CD45 expression, and monocyte-derived macrophages with high CD11b and high CD45 expression—but their accuracy has been questionable. Recently, researchers have attempted to track the development of these two types of cells in normal mice using new genetic marker technologies, but the results are still uncertain.

TAMs exhibit two distinct phenotypes, the pro-inflammatory M1 phenotype and the immunosuppressive M2 phenotype, which are regulated by factors in the tumor microenvironment. In the presence of inflammatory signals, microglia and macrophages are classically activated and develop an M1 phenotype, which enhances phagocyte migration, phagocytosis, and cytokine secretion. They also express MHC class II molecules and costimulatory molecules to promote T-cell activation. However, in the glioma state, especially in the advanced stages of tumor progression, TAMs polarize to the M2 phenotype, exhibit an immunosuppressive role, and promote tumor growth and invasion. It is important to note that the classification of M1 and M2 does not simply divide the role of TAMs into two. In the process of tumorigenesis and development, with the changes in immune microenvironment, M1 and M2 phenotypes can transform into each other, which is a dynamic process to balance the function of pro-inflammation/antitumor and anti-inflammation/pro-tumor.

TAMs are recruited to the tumor region by glioma-secreted chemokines such as CCL2, CCL7, CX3CL1, and stromal cell-derived factor-11 (SDF-1) and subsequently activated by glioma-derived growth factors such as colony-stimulating factor-1 (CSF-1), granulocyte-colony stimulating factor (G-CSF), and HGF. TAMs promote tumor growth and invasion by secreting matrix metalloproteinases and tumor cell proliferation-promoting factors such as EGF and VEGF. Under the influence of related cytokines, TAMs can further upregulate PD-L1, thereby promoting T-cell dysfunction. At the same time, the expression of FasL was upregulated, thereby promoting the apoptosis of T cells. In addition, glioma tissue induces a significant decrease in the expression of MHC molecules and pro-inflammatory cytokines (TNF-α) in TAMs, while increasing the expression of the transcription factor STAT3. Activation of STAT3 in TAMs promotes the secretion of the immunosuppressive cytokines IL-6 and IL-10, thereby suppressing the function of cytotoxic T lymphocytes.

Immunotherapy targeting the immunosuppressive activity of TAMs has been the focus of researchers. The transcription factor STAT3 is significantly upregulated in glioma-associated microglia and is therefore considered a viable target for immunotherapy. In vitro and in vivo experiments have demonstrated that knockdown of STAT3 by siRNA downregulates the secretion of immunosuppressive cytokines IL-6 and IL-10. The STAT3 inhibitors corosolic acid and oleanolic acid have also been shown to reduce the expression of CD163, a surface marker of M2 macrophages, and to downregulate IL-10 secretion, suggesting that these molecules may contribute to the conversion of M2 microglia to M1 type.

Myeloid-derived suppressor cells (MDSCs): MDSCs, a subpopulation of myeloid-derived cells, possess highly immunosuppressive activity that is distinct from the phenotype of TAMs. They accumulate in various sites, including tumors, blood, lymph nodes, or bone marrow, in response to cytokines secreted by the tumor, such as IL-6, IL-10, PGE2, TGF-β2, and VEGFβ. MDSCs are generally classified into two types: monocyte-derived MDSCs (M-MDSC) and granulocyte-derived MDSCs (G-MDSC). G-MDSCs are more immunosuppressive than M-MDSCs, as they can produce reactive oxygen species (ROS) to downregulate the expression of Bcl-2 on the surface of CD8+ T cells and trigger T-cell apoptosis. In contrast, M-MDSCs promote L-arginine metabolism through NO and Arg-1 pathways, leading to microenvironmental arginine depletion and ultimately, cell cycle arrest in T cells. Additionally, MDSCs induce NK cell and T-cell dysfunction while promoting the activation and expansion of Treg.

Studies have reported elevated G-MDSCs and M-MDSCs in the peripheral blood of GBM patients compared to healthy controls, with G-MDSCs being predominant in glioma tissues. This finding may have important implications for the targeted therapy of MDSCs. In a separate study, GL261 glioma model mice infused with GFP + CD11b + splenic monocytes had shorter survival time, faster tumor progression, and higher levels of MDSCs both intratumoral and in peripheral blood than control mice. Moreover, 30–50% of the detected MDSCs were GFP+, indicating that MDSCs may be derived from mononuclear cells. With the deepening of research on MDSCs, its targeted immunotherapy has attracted more attention. Various mouse glioma models have shown that inhibition of COX-2 expression, antibody-mediated immune depletion, and CCL2 neutralizing antibody to reduce the expression of MDSCs can prolong the survival of tumor-bearing mice.

5.5 Hypoxia and the Glioma Microenvironment

Hypoxia is a common phenomenon in tumors, which can lead to a series of consequences, such as abnormal vascularization, cytokine secretion, activation of oncogenes, and inactivation of tumor suppressor genes. Tumor cells adapt to hypoxic environments by undergoing changes such as proliferation, invasion, and metastasis. Tumors exposed to hypoxic microenvironments are often more invasive, exhibit higher malignant tendencies, and are prone to resistance to radiotherapy and chemotherapy, ultimately affecting patient prognosis.

It has been demonstrated that hypoxia has a significant effect on the generation of GSCs. As the intratumoral pH gradually drops below 6.5, non-glioma stem cells will upregulate their stemness-related genes and exhibit potential traits such as accelerated growth and increased tumorigenicity. Tumor cell proliferation in vitro cultures is limited by glucose availability, leading to the use of supraphysiological glucose concentrations in experiments. The addition of metabolic factors such as glucose plus lactate can significantly improve the phenotype of tumor cells, creating a culture environment similar to real hypoxia and acid stress.

Hypoxia promotes angiogenesis and radioresistance, both of which are characteristics of GSCs. The negative impact of hypoxia on patient survival may be partly explained by the increase in GSCs. The level of glioma invasion is significantly increased under hypoxic conditions, which may be related to HIF-1α. Knockdown of HIF-1α by shRNA significantly reduced the in vitro migration of GBM cells and their invasive ability in vivo. ACCA, a small molecule inhibitor of lactate transport, effectively reduced the invasive ability of GBM cells, and in vivo experiments confirmed that it prolonged the survival of GBM rats. HIF-1α-induced transcriptional genes such as calmodulin, VEGF, and other proteins stimulate blood vessel formation and provide nutrient delivery to tumor cells.

Vascullogenic Mimicry (VM) formation is a type of tumor adaptation to hypoxia. The HIF-1α-NRP-1 pathway or Bcl-2-dependent calcineurin overexpression promotes VM formation under hypoxic conditions. During VM formation in glioma, the expression of the vascular-endothelial-cadherin (CDH5) is regulated by HIF-1α and HIF-2α. As the oxygen concentration decreases in the tumor microenvironment, the expression of HIFs increases, inducing the multiple expression of CDH5, which in turn promotes VM formation through the interaction of β-catenin, PI3K, and VEGFR-2. Our study demonstrated that the expression of HIF-1α and epithelial-mesenchymal transition (EMT) markers in the tumor tissues of patients with recurrent glioma treated with bevacizumab was significantly higher than that in the non-treatment group. This finding indicated that the use of bevacizumab could exacerbate the hypoxia of glioma tissues. Moreover, glioma tissues' proliferation and invasion ability in the treatment group significantly increased. These phenomena disappeared after HIF-1α knockdown, which reaffirms the role of hypoxia in the induction of chemoresistance. This partly explains why bevacizumab-based chemotherapy regimens for glioma do not prolong patient survival, although they can reduce edema and improve clinical symptoms by reducing blood vessel permeability. These studies provide new targets and references for chemotherapy regimens in glioma.

5.6 Interactions in the Brain Tumor Microenvironment

In the previous sections, we described the main types of cells and cytokines in the glioma microenvironment and their roles in glioma progression. These interactions include the communication between tumor cells and supporting cells in the tumor stroma, the interaction between tumor cells and endothelial cells, and the interaction between tumor cells and immune cells (as discussed in Sect. 5.4, "The Immune Microenvironment of Glioma Is Unique"). This paragraph will focus on the interactions between tumor cells and supporting cells or endothelial cells.

In the glioma stroma, microglia and astrocytes are two important supporting cells that play a crucial role in the progression of glioma by maintaining the morphology of the tumor tissue and promoting tumor invasion. Intercellular communication between microglia and glioma cells has been shown to promote invasion by secreting inactive MMP-2 precursor proteins, which are activated by cytokines secreted by glioma cells, and mediate the degradation of ECM. Furthermore, microglia can upregulate TGF-β by secreting IL-1β, and TGF-β expression promotes angiogenesis, tumor proliferation, and tumor invasion by upregulating VEGF expression. Similarly, the interaction between astrocytes and tumor cells also plays a significant role in glioma invasion. Studies have shown that astrocyte-tumor cell interactions can upregulate MMP-2 expression. Co-culture of glioma cells and astrocytes demonstrated that overexpression of MMP-2 precursor in glioma cells enhanced tumor invasion, which was mediated by the uPA-plasminogen cascade. Glioma cells produced high levels of MMP-2 precursor protein and uPA and uPA receptors, and glioma cells produced fibrinogen, which was cleaved to active fibrinolytic enzymes and MMP-2 precursor protein to active MMP-2. High fibrinogen concentrations were also found in glioma sections, suggesting that a similar reaction may exist in human glioma tissue.

A surge of preclinical and clinical evidence in the past two decades has begun to elucidate the nervous system's role in promoting cancer growth. In light of the many mechanisms of tumor–nerve crosstalk and their accompanying clinicopathological ramifications, there are six broad avenues of intervention: inhibiting tumor growth, combating treatment resistance and tumor adaptation to stress, enhancing antitumor immunity, preventing dissemination and metastasis, and managing morbidity by dampening electrical hyperactivity and seizures as well as neuropathic pain. The nascent field of cancer neuroscience is growing rapidly, with parallel efforts in uncovering the mechanistic underpinnings of tumor–nerve interactions and developing novel therapies through collaborative academic and commercial efforts. Lessons learned from the tumor microenvironment suggest that disrupting tumor–nerve dialogue could eventually become a mainstay of clinical oncology, akin to anti-angiogenic and immunomodulatory therapies nowadays.

The glioma microenvironment is composed of various cell types, including endothelial cells, which secrete soluble cytokines such as brain-derived neurotrophic factor and VEGF that promote glioma cell proliferation and differentiation of GSCs. Additionally, endothelial cells can influence glioma (stem) cell functions in different ways. For instance, endothelial cells express NO synthase, which synthesizes NO and activates the Notch pathway in tumor stem cells, promoting self-renewal. Moreover, DLL4, a Notch pathway ligand, is highly expressed in glioma and endothelial cells in mouse glioma tissues, activating the Notch pathway and promoting tumor angiogenesis. Tumor endothelial cells also maintain the undifferentiated phenotype of cancer stem cells via Shh activation of the Hedgehog pathway in glioma. These interactions create a complex network of glioma progression, and it is essential to study the roles of multiple factors together, rather than in isolation and one-sidedly.

Further Reading

Bloch O, Crane CA, Kaur R, et al. Gliomas promote immunosuppression through induction of B7-H1 expression in tumor-associated macrophages. Clin Cancer Res. 2013;19(12):3165–75.

Cai JJ, Qi ZX, Hua W, et al. Increased expression of Capn4 is associated with the malignancy of human glioma. CNS Neurosci Ther. 2014;20(6):521–7.

Cai JJ, Qi ZX, Chen LC, et al. miR-124 suppresses the migration and invasion of glioma cells in vitro via Capn4. Oncol Rep. 2016;35(1):284–90.

Candolfi M, Curtin JF, Yagiz K, et al. B cells are critical to T-cell-mediated antitumor immunity induced by a combined immune-stimulatory/conditionally cytotoxic therapy for glioblastoma. Neoplasia. 2011;13(10):947–60.

Charles N, Ozawa T, Squatrito M, et al. Perivascular nitric oxide activates notch signaling and promotes stem-like character in PDGF-induced glioma cells. Cell Stem Cell. 2010;6(2):141–52.

Fujiwara Y, Komohara Y, Ikeda T, et al. Corosolic acid inhibits glioblastoma cell proliferation by suppressing the activation of signal transducer and activator of transcription-3 and nuclear factor-kappa B in tumor cells and tumor-associated macrophages. Cancer Sci. 2011;102(1):206–11.

Glass R, Synowitz M. CNS macrophages and peripheral myeloid cells in brain tumours. Acta Neuropathol. 2014;128(3):347–62.

Jarry U, Jeannin P, Pineau L, et al. Efficiently stimulated adult microglia cross-prime naive CD8+ T cells injected in the brain. Eur J Immunol. 2013;43(5):1173–84.

Jin X, Jin X, Sohn YW, et al. Blockade of EGFR signaling promotes glioma stem-like cell invasiveness by abolishing ID3-mediated inhibition of p27(KIP1) and MMP3 expression. Cancer Lett. 2013;328(2):235–42.

Monje M, Borniger JC, D'Silva NJ, et al. Roadmap for the emerging field of cancer neuroscience. Cell. 2020;181(2):219–22.

Shi DD, Guo JA, Hoffman HI, et al. Therapeutic avenues for cancer neuroscience: translational frontiers and clinical opportunities. Lancet Oncol. 2022;23(2):e62–74.

Talasila KM, Soentgerath A, Euskirchen P, et al. EGFR wild-type amplification and activation promote invasion and development of glioblastoma independent of angiogenesis. Acta Neuropathol. 2013;125(5):683–98.

Verhaak RG, Hoadley KA, Purdom E, et al. Integrated genomic analysis identifies clinically relevant subtypes of glioblastoma characterized by abnormalities in PDGFRA, IDH1, EGFR, and NF1. Cancer Cell. 2010;17(1):98–110.

Wainwright DA, Chang AL, Dey M, et al. Durable therapeutic efficacy utilizing combinatorial blockade against IDO, CTLA-4, and PD-L1 in mice with brain tumors. Clin Cancer Res. 2014;20(20):5290–301.

Xu H, Rahimpour S, Nesvick CL, et al. Activation of hypoxia signaling induces phenotypic transformation of glioma cells: implications for bevacizumab antiangiogenic therapy. Oncotarget. 2015;6(14):11882–93.

Zhang M, Kleber S, Rohrich M, et al. Blockade of TGF-β signaling by the TGFβR-I kinase inhibitor LY2109761 enhances radiation response and prolongs survival in glioblastoma. Cancer Res. 2011;71(23):7155–67.

Zhao Y, Xiao A, Dipierro CG, et al. An extensive invasive intracranial human glioblastoma xenograft model: role of high level matrix metalloproteinase 9. Am J Pathol. 2010;176(6):3032–49.

Advances in Genomics and Epigenetics of Glioma

6

Hui Yang and Lingchao Chen

Malignant gliomas are the most treatment-resistant cancers in the central nervous system. In recent years, genome-wide molecular-profiling studies, including exome sequencing and DNA methylation microarray, have revealed the characteristic genetic alterations and epigenetic profiles in different types of gliomas. As mentioned earlier, GBM was classified into three groups based on molecular characteristics: proneuronal, classical, and mesenchymal. Further, many studies showed that IDH1/IDH2 mutations, 1p/19q deletions, and TERTp mutations are important biomarkers for glioma classification. They could improve the prediction of patient outcomes and guide individualized treatment. Herein, we highlight the developments of the molecular genetics and epigenetics, including gene mutations, methylation, histone modifications, noncoding RNA, and other epigenetic insights in gliomas. We also reviewed the current landscape of biomarkers used in this disease. Novel approaches to the genetic and epigenetic characterization of gliomas based on large-scale DNA-methylation profiling and next-generation sequencing are also discussed. It provides an overview of how these advances will help clinicians gain deep understanding of glioma development and provide new ideas for precision therapies.

H. Yang · L. Chen (✉)
Department of Neurosurgery, Huashan Hospital, Fudan University, Shanghai, China

6.1 New Mutations in Glioma

In the past few years, a number of gene mutations in gliomas have been identified, and these mutations not only help clinicians to more accurately assess patient prognosis but also provide new directions for researchers to elucidate the pathogenesis of gliomas.

EGFR, a member of the ErbB receptor complex kinase family, has been widely studied in gliomas. EGFR amplification is found in 40% of glioblastomas, with half of these tumors harboring genetic rearrangement of EGFR exons 2–7. This aberration leads to the expression of EGFRvIII, which is constitutively activated by the lack of extracellular ligand-binding region. However, current therapies against EGFR have not significantly improved OS in glioblastoma patients. Therefore, scientists continue to work on new antibodies, vaccines, RNA-based therapies, and combinations of signaling pathway inhibitors to treat these patients with EGFR mutation.

IDH mutation is the early genetic event that occurs during the development of glioma. The WHO 2021 formalizes IDH mutation as a molecular biomarker of adult astrocytomas and oligodendrogliomas. IDH mutation induces a

Y. Mao (ed.), *Progress in the Diagnosis and Treatment of Gliomas*, Experts' Perspectives on Medical Advances, https://doi.org/10.1007/978-981-99-0123-4_6

neomorphic enzymatic activity, which can convert alpha-ketoglutarate into D-2-hydroxyglutarate (2-HG). Accumulation of 2-HG leads to significant epigenetic changes in glioma, altering methylation of histones and DNA. Increased DNA methylation and gene silencing genome-widely induced by 2-HG are often referred to the G-CIMP, which promotes tumorigenesis through repression of cell differentiation. Current studies clearly suggest that IDH mutation is a better prognosis biomarker.

CIC is a member of the high mobility group (HMG)-box superfamily of transcriptional repressors. CIC mutation can repress RTK-induced gene expression and increase pro-survival and proliferative transcriptional profiles. FUBP1 is a key regulator of tumor suppressor and oncogene alternative splicing. FUBP1 loss leads to widespread alterations in RNA splicing and increased MYC transcript levels. Mutations in CIC and FUBP1 occur in oligodendrogliomas at rates as high as 60% and 30%, respectively. Intriguingly, the genomic localization of CIC and FUBP1, on chromosomes 19q and 1p, respectively, is consistent with the notion that 1p/19q codeletion partially disables key tumor suppressors resident on the 1p and 19q chromosomal arms in oligodendrogliomas.

ATRX is a protein of SWI/SNF, which is an ATP-dependent transcriptional regulator, used to maintain telomere homeostasis. Mutations in this gene are associated with X-linked syndromes exhibiting cognitive disabilities as well as alpha-thalassemia syndrome. These mutations have been shown to cause global DNA methylation, which may provide a link between chromatin remodeling, DNA methylation, and gene expression in developmental processes. Cells deficient in ATRX undergo p53-dependent cell death, which partially explains the co-occurrence of ATRX and TP53 mutations in glioma. Further, patients with ATRX-deficient, IDH-mutant, non-co-deleted astrocytoma have a better prognosis than those with ATRX-intact, IDH-mutant, non-co-deleted. Beyond their abnormal genomic and epigenomic phenotypes, ATRX-deficient glioma display lengthening of telomeres via alternative lengthening of telomeres (ALT). Thus, ATRX mutations may define a subclass of IDH1 mutant astrocytomas, which is associated with better prognosis.

Recent studies have shown a close relationship between genomics and epigenetics in gliomagenesis. For example, encoding the histone variant H3.3 plays a central role in transcription regulation, DNA repair, DNA replication, and chromosomal stability. H3F3A mutations occur in 70–80% of childhood gliomas, especially diffuse pontine gliomas. H3F3A mutations contained two major types: (1) K27M and (2) G34R/V. K27M is located at the caudal end of H3.3. H3K27M gliomas often occur at midline locations. However, H3F3AG34R/V occurs in the hemispheres of the brain and tends to develop in older individuals. These findings suggest that K27M and G34R/V are specific in terms of tumor location and age. H3K27M causes global reduction of cellular histone H3 lysine 27 trimethylation via impaired recruitment of polycomb repressive complex 2 (PRC2) and inhibition of EZH2. Besides, H3K27M gliomas frequently harbor mutations in TP53 and/or PPM1D and amplification of proto-oncogenes, such as PDGFRA, MYC, MYCN, CDK4, CDK6, and CCND1–3. Hemispheric malignant gliomas in children comprise different molecular subgroups, including H3F3A-G34-mutant tumors and a small fraction of IDH-mutant glioblastomas.

In addition to mutations and amplifications, a number of aberrant fusion genes have been detected in gliomas. The most representative of these fusions is the BRAF gene fusion, which is almost exclusively found in fibrous astrocytomas. Another abnormal alteration of BRAF is the BRAFV600E mutation, which can be used to identify fibrous astrocytomas, and high-grade astrocytomas.

The incidence of fusion genes in gliomas has been suggested to be high in pleomorphic yellow astrocytomas and GBM. In addition, RNA sequencing data have revealed several fusion genes in malignant gliomas. The two most obvious fusion genes are FGFR (FGFR1-TACC1 and FGFR3-TACC3) and EGFR (EGFR-SEPT and EGFR-PSPH). The former is present in 3% of

GBMs, and the latter is seen in about 8% of GBMs. These alterations have been considered to be new drug targets, offering new hope for future interventions. In China, Jiang's team described the discovery of MET 14exon skipping (METex14) in secondary glioblastoma (sGBM). They also showed PTPRZ1-MET(ZM) fusion gene could promote the malignant progression of glioma. Based on the mechanism of ZM fusion, their team initiated a phase I clinical trial of the MET inhibitor PLB-1001 (Beritinib) for the treatment of HGG, providing a new treatment strategy for patients with this type.

The newly discovered single-gene mutation adds to the complexity and molecular heterogeneity of glioma. It will prompt a shift from the traditional-pathological classification to a new view that combines histological and molecular classification in order to better assess treatment response and clinical prognosis.

6.2 Altered Methylation in Gliomas

In gliomagenesis, alterations in gene expression are often associated with DNA methylation and epigenetic alterations of chromosomes. An example of clear clinical relevance is the methylation of the MGMT promoter. Approximately, 40% of IDH wild-type glioblastomas have hypermethylation of an MGMT-associated 5′ CpG island, which results in transcriptional repression and reduced MGMT expression. MGMT-promoter methylation has been closely linked with benefit of temozolomide therapy and prolonged survival of patients with glioblastoma. MGMT methylation can be detected by pyrophosphate sequencing and methylation-specific MSP-PCR techniques, which are now widely used in clinics. The specificity of immunohistochemical staining for MGMT methylation is relatively low.

The TCGA project in gliomas has identified a large number of methylation events in the promoter regions of genes and has also demonstrated the complexity of DNA methylation patterns.

Four major subgroups of adult glioblastoma have been identified, including an IDH-mutant, G-CIMP-positive, and typically MGMT-promoter-methylated subgroup with a proneural gene-expression profile and three subgroups of IDH wild-type glioblastoma. Among the IDH wild-type glioblastoma subgroups, RTK I glioblastomas predominantly occur in adolescents and young adults and are characterized by PDGFRA amplification and a proneural gene-expression profile. The RTK II and the "mesenchymal" IDH-wild-type glioblastoma subtypes predominate in patients >50 years of age and are distinguished by different DNA-methylation profiles, as well as fewer copy-number aberrations and a mesenchymal gene-expression signature in mesenchymal glioblastoma.

Recent studies have shown that the TET family of proteins is not only involved in DNA demethylation but also plays an important epigenetic modifying role in the developmental process, and its aberrant expression can lead to methylation pattern disorders, which are closely associated with many cancers and developmental disorder syndromes. This modification process also requires the involvement of DNA methyltransferase DNMT3A and its family members. DNMT3A has a catalytic unit and a regulatory unit that regulates its own activity. The regulatory unit combines with the catalytic unit and inhibits its binding to DNA, keeping DNMT3A in a low-activity state and ensuring that DNMT3A does not establish methylation modifications on the genome at will. Currently, Professor Yanhui Xu and others from Fudan University have resolved the protein structures of DNMT3A and TET, and the future development of targeted drugs is no longer far away.

6.3 Histone Modifications in Gliomas

Histone modification (HM) takes place in several ways in the mammalian epigenome. The core histone possesses C-terminal as well as N-terminal attaching areas. Among these, the N-terminal is predominantly relevant, because the lysine moiety of the N-terminal expands outside the nucleosome and is easily reachable for modifications, such as methylation, acetylation, ADP ribosylation, phosphorylation, and ubiquitination. These modifications play a crucial role in altering gene expression without changing the base pairs.

The methylation of histones is widely studied and is generally performed by histone methyl transferase (HMT). The methylation of histones can occur on lysine and arginine residues, and lysine residues can be mono-, di-, or tri-methylated, while arginine residues are only mono- or di-methylated. Numerous studies have found that histone methyltransferases such as MLL1, MLL2, EZH2, and G9a control the methylation level of lysine situated in histone in glioma cells. These modifications are strongly connected with the regulation of gene transcription and genome integration. Protein arginine methyltransferase 5 (PRMT5) gene is also used for diagnosing and management of GBM. It has been found that GBM cells treated with the inhibitor of PRMT5 can induce apoptosis of differentiated GBM cells as well as drive undifferentiated primary patient-mediated glioma cells into a non-replicative senescence state.

Histone acetylation occurs at the more conserved N-terminal lysine position of H3 and H4 and is mainly regulated by histone acetyltransferases and histone deacetylases. Because of the large number of sites available for acetylation on nucleosomes, histone acetylation can be diverse; however, histone acetylation and deacetylation at specific gene sites occur in a site-specific, nonrandom manner. Acetylation may regulate gene transcription through its effects on histone charges and interacting proteins. Among these, deacetylase inhibitors are supposed to be the more promising novel drugs currently available for epigenetically targeted therapies. Among the diverse groups of HDAC enzymes, HDAC1, HDAC2, HDAC3, HDAC5, and HDAC9 have gone through substantial alterations in glioma cell lines. Furthermore, the levels of H3 acetylation are raised in high-grade astrocytoma. It is known that class II and IV HDACs are downregulated in GBM in comparison with low-grade astrocytomas and healthy brain tissues. HDACIs have also been applied for treating GBM in combination with chemotherapy and radiation therapy. Besides, the anticancer mode of action of HDACIs, such as stopping cell cycle and boosting cell differentiation, suppressing angiogenesis, and triggering apoptosis, can ultimately suppress the proliferation as well as programmed cell death of glioma cells.

In addition, it is worth mentioning that the PRC is an important gene regulator in embryonic development, in which PRC2 is responsible for catalyzing the methylation modification of H3K27 and plays an important role in the development and progression of many tumors, including glioma and ventricular meningioma. The expression of EZH2 is positively correlated with glioma grade and negatively correlated with prognosis, and the knockdown of EZH2 in vitro and in vivo can significantly inhibit glioma growth. In addition, some scholars have attempted to use inhibitors of epigenetic factors (EZH2 and BMI1) to treat glioma in situ in a mouse model, providing a new target site for the drug treatment of glioma.

6.4 Advances in the Study of Noncoding RNA in Glioma

Gliomas are regulated at the RNA level by various modalities, such as miRNA, long-stranded noncoding RNA (lncRNA), and small nucleolar RNA (snoRNA), which also influence tumor cell survival and other functions. miRNAs are a group of small RNA sequences that can inhibit mRNA transcription through complementary association with mRNAs, leading to decreased protein synthesis. miRNAs are currently known in the control of cell metabolism in GBM. Furthermore, miRNAs control metabolic gene expression directly or via the control of metabolism-associated oncogenes and tumor suppressor. Several miRNAs could target enzymes of mRNAs leading to metabolic processes, such as lipids, glucose and glutamine metabolism, glycolysis, and oxidative phosphorylation. Most miRNAs are situated in genes of glioma, and these genes can control around 3% of the whole genes and 30% of coding genes in glioma. Thus, one miRNA can probably affect 100 GBM mRNAs, while one mRNA can be regulated by different miRNAs. In GBM cells, many studies revealed that miRNA-181 was the most trusted marker in glioma diagnosis. It can directly target MGMT and downregulate its expression, which can improve the responsiveness of patients to TMZ in clinic. EGFR can be targeted by various miRNAs such as miR-128, miR-7, and miR-219-5p, which are downregulated in GBM. The oncogenic KRAS enhances cancer cell growth by dissociating the metabolism of glutamine and glucose. miR-9 affects KRAS indirectly by targeting neurofibromin 1 (KRAS inhibitor). Besides, overexpression of miR-9 occurs in GBM, and its expression is also linked with poor disease prognosis. Although miRNAs with oncogenic effects are of great importance for tumor therapy, they are limited by a lack of stability and inefficient delivery. Although viruses can be an effective delivery vector, they contain antigenic components that induce immune responses and damage the host chromosome. Some non-viral vectors, such as inorganic particles, liposomes, membrane-penetrating peptides, and cationic polymers, are currently less effective. In vitro experiments and animal models have shown that a novel nanocapsule-based miRNA delivery vector can effectively improve the stability and delivery efficiency of miRNA, thereby inhibiting tumor vasculature formation and tumor growth.

lncRNAs are noncoding transcripts of more than 200 nucleotides (200 nt), playing a pivotal role in the regulation of genes in cancer metabolism. It has been shown that 27 lncRNAs are upregulated, and 198 lncRNAs are downregulated in GBM, indicating the significant role in GBM. The lncRNA TP53TG1 assists cell migration and proliferation via the expression of genes like PKM2 and IDH1 in glioma cultures, in the presence of reduced glucose. The lncRNA LEF1-AS1 facilitates the multiplication of GBM cells and impedes apoptosis via the AKT/mTOR pathway, which controls glycolysis. However, more studies are needed to authenticate the link between lncRNAs and the regulation of GBM. In contrast, circular RNAs play a significant role in cellular metabolism in GBM. For example, the FBXW7circRNA translates a novel 21-kDa protein named FBXW7-185aa and lessens the USP28-mediated stabilization of c-Myc, which might be linked to the Warburg effect. Though not much is known regarding the management of cell metabolism by circRNAs.

6.5 Epigenetics Is Constantly Changing in the Development and Progression of Gliomas

Subtle changes in the balance between genomics and epigenetics can affect DNA repair, cell cycle regulation, and cell differentiation. If the balance is disturbed, the cell may undergo a malignant transformation. There is much evidence showing that epigenetic alterations in precursor/stem cell may be the early stage of cancerous transformation. One hypothesis shows that precursor/stem cells are in a stable state during the pre-tumor stage. Then, they undergo a series of epigenetic changes that eventually lead to cancerous transformation. During the development of glioma, epigenetic regulation might sensitize glial precursor/neural stem cells to decrease tumor suppressor expression or activate proto-oncogene expression. In the proneuronal type of GBM, G-CIMP and IDH mutations inhibit histone and DNA methylation, leading to the inactivation of tumor suppressor genes.

Another challenge is the recurrence of gliomas. However, it has been found that tumor progression is associated with genomic instability, demethylation, and some important oncogene alterations. Little is known about the genomic and epigenetic alterations in glioma recurrence. Therefore, it has been suggested that a paired analysis of primary and secondary GBM is needed in the future to better understand the mechanisms of tumor recurrence.

Molecular typing for individualized treatment of gliomas requires a comprehensive molecular/genetic analysis of the patient's tumor tissue. Although a large amount of molecular data on

GBM has been obtained from tumor tissue, little is known about the molecular characteristics of tumor-infiltrating marginal tissue. Infiltrating glioma cells can escape surgical resection and eventually lead to tumor recurrence. In the infiltrative margin, glioma cells are mixed with non-tumor cells, including neurons, oligodendrocytes, reactive astrocytes, and microglia. This feature poses a significant obstacle to molecular typing, and future studies may require the use of physical techniques to separate these cells, such as laser capture microscopy and cell sorting, although application to microscopy is still difficult. Since glial and neurons are tightly intertwined with surrounding cells, establishing a new method of extracting cell-specific molecular markers would be a breakthrough to help us better understand diffuse gliomas.

Some other advances in the life sciences include high-resolution chromatin folding, imaging, optogenetics, etc. The former allows for a more detailed understanding of the genetic characteristics of gliomas, while the latter allows for the use of light to control biological processes such as cell proliferation and apoptosis. Thus, tumor cells could be genetically engineered to be sensitive to light, allowing invisible "light knives" to be used to treat the remnants of tumors that cannot be removed intraoperatively. In addition, some algorithmic improvements will allow us to learn more about low-abundance mutations and genetic changes in noncoding regions of the tumor genome, opening another door to understanding tumor genomics and epigenetics.

As we gain a better understanding of glioma genomics and epigenetics, neuropathologists need to accelerate the pace at which molecular biological data can be integrated with routine diagnostic approaches. In past practice, several new biomarkers have been integrated into clinic, including MGMT methylation analysis, EGFR amplification and mutation, 1p/19q deletion, and IDH1/IDH2 mutations, which have effectively optimized neuro-oncology diagnostics and treatment. It is believed that as the cost of next-generation sequencing technology decreases, big data will be applied to pathology diagnosis and precisive treatment.

Further Reading

An Z, Aksoy O, Zheng T, et al. Epidermal growth factor receptor and EGFRvIII in glioblastoma: signaling pathways and targeted therapies. Oncogene. 2018;37(12):1561–75.

Baumgarten P, Harter PN, Tönjes M, et al. Loss of FUBP1 expression in gliomas predicts FUBP1 mutation and is associated with oligodendroglial differentiation, IDH1 mutation and 1p/19q loss of heterozygosity. Neuropathol Appl Neurobiol. 2014;40(2): 205–16.

Brennan CW, Verhaak RG, McKenna A, et al. The somatic genomic landscape of glioblastoma. Cell. 2013;155(2):462–77.

Chen CCL, Deshmukh S, Jessa S, et al. Histone H3.3G34-mutant interneuron progenitors co-opt PDGFRA for gliomagenesis. Cell. 2020;183(6):1617–1633.e22.

Chistiakov DA, Chekhonin IV, Chekhonin VP. The EGFR variant III mutant as a target for immunotherapy of glioblastoma multiforme. Eur J Pharmacol. 2017;810:70–82.

Chou FJ, Liu Y, Lang F, Yang C. D-2-Hydroxyglutarate in glioma biology. Cells. 2021;10(9):2345.

Dang L, Su SM. Isocitrate dehydrogenase mutation and (*R*)-2-hydroxyglutarate: from basic discovery to therapeutics development. Annu Rev Biochem. 2017;86:305–31.

Darabi S, Xiu J, Samec T, et al. Capicua (CIC) mutations in gliomas in association with MAPK activation for exposing a potential therapeutic target. Med Oncol. 2023;40(7):197.

El-Hashash AHK. Histone H3K27M mutation in brain tumors. Adv Exp Med Biol. 2021;1283:43–52.

Gencel-Augusto J, Bivona TG. Unlocking the EGFR-mediated epitranscriptome: a pathway to novel therapies. Mol Cell. 2023;83(23):4199–201.

Gusyatiner O, Hegi ME. Glioma epigenetics: from subclassification to novel treatment options. Semin Cancer Biol. 2018;51:50–8.

Haase S, Garcia-Fabiani MB, Carney S, et al. Mutant ATRX: uncovering a new therapeutic target for glioma. Expert Opin Ther Targets. 2018;22(7): 599–613.

Hu L, Li Z, Cheng J, et al. Crystal structure of TET2-DNA complex: insight into TET-mediated 5mC oxidation. Cell. 2013;155(7):1545–55.

Hu H, Mu Q, Bao Z, et al. Mutational landscape of secondary glioblastoma guides MET-targeted trial in brain tumor. Cell. 2018;175(6):1665–1678.e18.

Huse JT, Aldape KD. The evolving role of molecular markers in the diagnosis and management of diffuse glioma. Clin Cancer Res. 2014;20(22):5601–11.

Kohli RM, Zhang Y. TET enzymes, TDG and the dynamics of DNA demethylation. Nature. 2013;502(7472):472–9.

Lawrence M, Daujat S, Schneider R. Lateral thinking: how histone modifications regulate gene expression. Trends Genet. 2016;32(1):42–56.

Lin B, Ziebro J, Smithberger E, et al. EGFR, the Lazarus target for precision oncology in glioblastoma. Neuro Oncol. 2022;24(12):2035–62.

Liu I, Jiang L, Samuelsson ER, et al. The landscape of tumor cell states and spatial organization in H3-K27M mutant diffuse midline glioma across age and location. Nat Genet. 2022;54(12):1881–94.

Nandakumar P, Mansouri A, Das S. The role of ATRX in glioma biology. Front Oncol. 2017;7:236.

Nazem A, Lavezo J, Abdullaev Z, et al. Diffuse hemispheric glioma with H3-3B G34R mutation: expanding the spectrum of histone H3 genes in diffuse hemispheric glioma, H3 G34-mutant. J Neuropathol Exp Neurol. 2023;83(1):58–60.

Noll A, Myers C, Biery MC, et al. Therapeutic HDAC inhibition in hypermutant diffuse intrinsic pontine glioma. Neoplasia. 2023;43:100921.

Paskeh MDA, Mehrabi A, Gholami MH, et al. EZH2 as a new therapeutic target in brain tumors: molecular landscape, therapeutic targeting and future prospects. Biomed Pharmacother. 2022;146:112532.

Rezaei O, Honarmand K, Nateghinia S, et al. miRNA signature in glioblastoma: potential biomarkers and therapeutic targets. Exp Mol Pathol. 2020;117:104550.

Rolle K. miRNA multiplayers in glioma. from bench to bedside. Acta Biochim Pol. 2015;62(3): 353–65.

Sachamitr P, Ho JC, Ciamponi FE, et al. PRMT5 inhibition disrupts splicing and stemness in glioblastoma. Nat Commun. 2021;12(1):979.

Schreck KC, Langat P, Bhave VM, et al. Integrated molecular and clinical analysis of BRAF-mutant glioma in adults. NPJ Precis Oncol. 2023; 7(1):23.

Turkalp Z, Karamchandani J, Das S. IDH mutation in glioma: new insights and promises for the future. JAMA Neurol. 2014;71(10):1319–25.

Westphal M, Maire CL, Lamszus K. EGFR as a target for glioblastoma treatment: an unfulfilled promise. CNS Drugs. 2017;31(9):723–35.

Wierzbicki K, Ravi K, Franson A, et al. Targeting and therapeutic monitoring of H3K27M-mutant glioma. Curr Oncol Rep. 2020;22(2):19.

Xu X, Liang Y, Gareev I, et al. LncRNA as potential biomarker and therapeutic target in glioma. Mol Biol Rep. 2023;50(1):841–51.

You G, Fan X, Hu H, et al. Fusion genes altered in adult malignant gliomas. Front Neurol. 2021;12:715206.

7 Application of Multimodal Imaging Techniques in Diagnosis and Treatment of Glioma

Tianming Qiu and Jinsong Wu

7.1 The Role of Conventional Imaging Should Not Be Neglected

In recent years, several imaging methods have been developed for the diagnosis and differential diagnosis of glioma, such as diffusion tensor imaging (DTI), magnetic resonance spectroscopy (MRS), magnetic resonance perfusion weighted imaging (PWI), and positron emission computed tomography (PET-CT) or PET-MR. Although these new methods are valuable, conventional imaging remains the most important technique. The fundamental imaging characteristics of glioma, including its origin, growth, infiltration of tumor cells, pathophysiological features, and response to treatment, are determined by these factors, and conventional imaging can provide important information for their assessment.

When diagnosing glioma based on imaging, it is essential to consider the patient's clinical presentation, neurological examination, and laboratory tests. Multimodality imaging should take into account the location of the lesion (intra/extracerebral), the number of lesions (single/multiple), the growth characteristics of the lesion (infiltrative/swelling/atrophic), and the internal texture of the lesion. While new imaging techniques such as DTI, MRS, PWI, PET, and others are important, this section emphasizes the value of routine cranial CT and MRI sequences in the diagnosis of glioma. Further discussion of these advanced imaging methods will be presented in other chapters.

Gliomas typically appear as isointense or hypointense masses with poorly defined borders on CT. In cases where there is bleeding or calcification, they may appear as high-density lesions. When intracranial tumor apoplexy is suspected, enhanced CT can help differentiate between a tumor and clarify its borders. On T1-weighted (T1W) imaging, gliomas appear as iso- or low-signal, while they appear as high-signal on T2-weighted (T2W) imaging. Fluid attenuation inversion recovery (FLAIR) sequences are more sensitive in detecting lesions and displaying their boundaries, making it the first choice for showing low-grade gliomas. Diffusion-weighted imaging (DWI) can help distinguish inflammation from a tumor. Gliomas typically have a slightly higher signal on DWI than inflammation because the cell density in inflammatory lesions is much lower than that in tumors. In brain abscesses, the limited diffusion of water molecules inside often results in a higher DWI signal, which can be distinguished from the necrotic component in high-grade gliomas (HGG). Irregular peripheral enhancement is often suggestive of HGG, where necrosis or cystic lesions are present. The inner walls of the enhancing foci are often heteroge-

T. Qiu · J. Wu (✉)
Department of Neurosurgery, Huashan Hospital, Fudan University, Shanghai, China

Y. Mao (ed.), *Progress in the Diagnosis and Treatment of Gliomas*, Experts' Perspectives on Medical Advances, https://doi.org/10.1007/978-981-99-0123-4_7

neous, unlike brain abscesses. It should be noted that some HGGs may have no significant enhancement or only scattered enhancement, while a few benign gliomas, such as pilocytic astrocytoma, may also show significant enhancement. Enhanced T1 imaging is currently the preferred sequence for determining borders in HGGs.

It is important to note that in most cases, anatomical structures and gray-white matter boundaries do not appear within the tumor on conventional MRI. However, in rare cases, there may be significant anatomical structures within the tumor. For instance, within insula and basal ganglia gliomas, distinct anatomical distribution of the lentiform nucleus, external capsule, nucleus claustralis, extreme capsule, and insula cortex can be seen, even though these anatomical structures exhibit relatively high abnormal T2 signals on MRI. At this point, the diagnosis of glioma cannot be easily ruled out.

7.2 Magnetic Resonance Spectroscopy Is Valuable for the Diagnosis of Glioma

The ability to differentiate between tumor and non-neoplastic lesions is crucial in formulating treatment strategies. Magnetic resonance spectroscopy (MRS) has been an important method for analyzing lesion metabolism, and its clinical value has gradually become evident. MRS has advanced from single voxel to multiple voxels, from two-dimensional imaging to three-dimensional reconstruction, from detecting a few single compounds to quantitatively and synergistically detecting multiple indicators and from preoperative diagnosis to postoperative follow-up.

Currently, MRS plays a significant role in the perioperative management of glioma. Firstly, the choline/*N*-acetylaspartate (Cho/NAA) ratio has been used as an important reference for the diagnosis. In our previous studies comparing this ratio with the pathology of glioma, we found that the probability of determining the lesion as HGG was 38%, 60%, 79%, and 90% when the ratio was 0.5, 1.0, 1.5, and 2.0, respectively. The probability of LGG was 16%, 39%, 67%, and 87%, respectively. Therefore, the Cho/NAA ratio cannot only help us to diagnose glioma but also be used to outline the metabolic boundary for tumor resection. Secondly, after adjuvant therapy, MRS could be utilized to differentiate whether the enhancement on structural imaging is recurrence or pseudo-progression of glioma. Recently, it has been reported that the mean Cho/NAA ratio in the recurrent tumor is 2.72 and in the radiation necrosis is 1.46 ($p < 0.01$); the choline/lipid (Cho/lipid) ratio in recurrent tumor is 2.78 and in radiation necrosis is 0.6. Again, since IDH mutations are significantly associated with 2-HG, it was reported in 2012 on Nature Medicine that MRS can detect 2-HG. Elevated 2-HG concentrations were also detected in 2-HG-positive tumor specimens detected by MRS, confirming the correlation between such 2-HG-elevated tumors and IDH-1 or IDH-2 mutations. The correlation between tumors with elevated 2-HG concentrations and IDH-1 or IDH-2 gene mutations was also confirmed. The availability of 2-HG detection by MRS has brought the diagnosis of glioma to the protein and even gene level. Finally, the use of multivoxel 3D MRS provides a more reliable basis for target selection for puncture biopsy of intracerebral lesions. In the case of an undiagnosed intracerebral lesion, the metabolic images of MRS can be used as a reference for target selection when performing image-guided needle biopsy, thus making the procedure more precise and having a better chance of obtaining reliable pathological results.

However, when using MRS for the diagnosis and differential diagnosis of glioma, it is important to know that: (1) the existing MRS technology is inherently unstable, especially when the lesion is close to the skull base, around the ventricles, or under the tentorium. When using MRS, the stability of the baseline should be determined first (2). MRS can be used to help differentiate tumors from non-tumor lesions, but not the degree of benignity or malignancy of the tumor neither the exact pathology nor the grade of glioma. Therefore, the prerequisite for using it to diagnose glioma is structural imaging, and MRS has its value only based on structural images (3). When using MRS to identify recurrent glioma and pseudo-progression, it is necessary to combine it with the patient's clinical manifestations, structural images of enhanced MRI, magnetic resonance perfusion imaging, amino acid PET, etc., rather than only relying on MRS result to make a judgment and guide treatment. Some inflammatory lesions (especially inflammatory demyelinating lesions) may show a significant increase in Cho and a decrease in NAA.

7.3 To Evaluate Tumor Perfusion by "Relative Cerebral Blood Volume"

PWI has become increasingly utilized for observing blood perfusion in intracranial lesions. It can aid in preoperative diagnosis and differential diagnosis of glioma, target selection during glioma needle biopsy, and differentiation between glioma recurrence and radiation necrosis.

Relative cerebral blood volume (rCBV) is a measurement based on a comparison of the lesion with normal brain tissue. There are two methods of comparison, one comparing the lesion with normal brain tissue in the mirror image of the lesion and the other comparing the lesion with normal white matter areas of the brain; the advantages and disadvantages of which are still inconclusive. In practice, rCBV is used (1) to distinguish tumors from non-tumorigenic lesions, but it is also used to distinguish other tumors that also show enhancement, such as HGG from CNS lymphoma. The parenchyma of the HGG is often characterized by high perfusion due to its abundance of neovascularization, while lymphoma is composed of dense lymphoma cells and lack of vascularization, thus showing hypoperfusion compared with gliomas. rCBV is also used (2) to distinguish recurrent glioma from pseudo-progressive tumor. The former shows high perfusion due to the recurrence of the tumor with massive neovascularization, while the latter shows low perfusion due to mainly radioactive necrotic tissue. Lastly, it is used (3) to distinguish HGG from brain metastasis. HGG has peritumoral edema with massive infiltration of tumor cells, and the rCBV of peritumoral tissue is often elevated. For brain metastasis, peritumor edema is due to cytotoxicity with no blood supply; therefore, the rCBV of the peritumor tissue is not high.

There are currently three methods of perfusion-weighted imaging (PWI) used in the diagnosis of glioma. These include T2-based dynamic susceptibility contrast (DSC), which reflects the neovascularization of the lesion; T1-based dynamic contrast-enhanced perfusion imaging (DCE), which reflects the vascular permeability of the lesion; and arterial spin labeling without contrast (ASL), which is increasingly used because it can remove the effect of contrast leakage compared with DSC. The optimal application of PWI for glioma diagnosis requires further research.

7.4 DTI Is an Important Tool for Preoperative Assessment of Subcortical Pathways

Brain function relies not only on the cortex but also on the integrity of subcortical pathways such as the pyramidal tracts, arcuate fasciculus, optic radiations, and others. It is therefore essential to accurately observe the relationship between fibers and tumors before glioma surgery. Tractography based on diffusion tensor imaging (DTI) can assist neurosurgeons in understanding the anatomy of fiber tracts during surgery and devising appropriate surgical approaches. An increasing number of studies have been conducted to validate the reliability of fibers shown by DTI through subcortical electrical stimulation. In our study, the DTI-displayed pyramidal tracts were about 8 mm from the positive site, with a sensitivity and specificity of over 90%. In another study, DTI indicated an 80% overlap between the language pathway and positive subcortical electrical stimulation sites, with a distance of approximately 6 mm. The distance between the visual pathway and subcortical electrical stimulation has not been reported yet, but animal studies have indicated a strong correlation between the visual pathway and the tracts shown by DTI. As white matter dissection techniques improve and our understanding of language networks and pathways grows, more studies have focused on the subdivision of different fibers within the language network using DTI. These include the uncinate fasciculus, inferior frontal-occipital fasciculus, superior longitudinal fasciculus (with different segments), arcuate fasciculus, frontal oblique fasciculus, and inferior longitudinal fasciculus, among others. DTI-based reconstruction of these fibers can be effectively integrated into the navigation of glioma surgery. This not only helps neurosurgeons better understand the relationship between the tumor and language fibers but also provides crucial technical support for subcortical electrical stimulation to verify and study the actual function of these pathways, thereby deepening our scientific understanding of the language network.

Due to the characteristics of fibers and the way tumors grow, few fibers pass through tumor tissues. In our previous experience with tractography, we were unable to trace fibers when the seed point was located within the tumor parenchyma. However, in the periphery of the tumor, fibers were often observed to wrap around the tumor or connect to a distant location, which helped us distinguish between tumor and non-tumor lesions. Furthermore, several studies have proposed using anisotropic scores to identify gliomas.

It is important to note that DTI-based tractography is subject to several factors that can influence its accuracy, such as scanning parameters, post-processing methods, threshold settings, and seed point selection. Therefore, while this technique provides valuable insights into the relationship between lesions and fibers, it should not be solely relied upon to determine the extent of resection in glioma surgery. Subcortical electrical stimulation remains the current gold standard for identifying motor or language pathways. Recent advances in multi-direction scanning, multi-*b*-value method, and diffusion spectrum imaging hold promise for providing more precise information for the study of neurofibers.

7.5 Resting-State BOLD Is a Useful Complement to Task-State BOLD for Preoperative Eloquent Area Localization

Safe glioma surgery requires precise functional brain localization to minimize postoperative disability. The blood oxygenation level-dependent (BOLD) technique is an important imaging method for preoperative brain localization. Numerous studies have demonstrated the effectiveness of BOLD imaging based on motor and language tasks in localizing functional areas, which correspond well with intraoperative electrical cortical stimulation results. However, BOLD acquisition and imaging cannot be performed when the patient has a preoperative neurological deficit or cannot cooperate with the task. Resting-state BOLD technology has recently been used to localize brain functions, which does not require patient cooperation and can acquire multiple functional areas by one-time scanning. Currently, the functional connectivity method and independent component analysis method are the two primary data processing methods of resting-state BOLD applied to preoperative localization in neurosurgery, with the functional connectivity method being relatively stable and reliable. In our recent study, functional connectivity-based resting BOLD localization showed good matching with conventional motor BOLD localization in motor areas, with sensitivity and specificity of 90.91% and 89.41%, respectively. Although resting BOLD does not show significant advantages over conventional speech BOLD in localizing speech areas, it is still an important complementary tool for preoperative speech localization in patients who cannot cooperate with BOLD scans for speech tasks. The advantage of resting BOLD is that it does not require patient cooperation, which allows us to use this technique to localize brain function in patients under general anesthesia. In our previous study, the sensitivity and specificity of resting BOLD in locating motor areas, with the aid of high-field intraoperative MRI, were 61.7% and

93.7%, respectively. This allows for real-time, noninvasive intraoperative functional brain localization and reduces the potential of seizures due to electrical stimulation.

Both resting BOLD and task BOLD are MRI techniques that indirectly measure neuronal activity by detecting changes in blood oxygenation levels. Therefore, caution must be exercised in the acquisition, analysis, and interpretation of the data as they may lead to misinterpretation of the results. While resting-state BOLD is a noninvasive, relatively reliable, simple, and fast method for preoperative brain localization in glioma surgery, it should be used in conjunction with task-based BOLD imaging for more comprehensive results. The two methods can complement each other, guiding more targeted intraoperative cortical stimulation, reducing the incidence of seizures due to electrical stimulation, and providing the neurosurgeon with a better understanding of the relationship between the eloquent area and the lesion. Further advancements in BOLD imaging technology are expected to improve the precision of glioma surgery.

7.6 PET Imaging Using Various Radiopharmaceutical Agents Is a Valuable Tool in the Diagnosis of Glioma

With the continuous development of PET technology, an increasing number of imaging agents are being used in clinical practice to aid in the diagnosis of glioma. The traditional theory of ^{18}F-FDG (^{18}F-fluorodeoxyglucose) is based on the fact that tumor glucose metabolism is higher than that of the surrounding normal tissue. However, in LGG, tumor glucose metabolism may not be higher than that of normal brain tissue, which can result in a false-negative result. Amino acid imaging agents, such as ^{11}C-methionine (^{11}C-MET), are better for glioma imaging because their uptake by cells is mainly related to the distribution of amino acid transporters on the cell surface and the metabolism of amino acids. Since brain tissue does not use methionine as a source of energy and has low uptake, it is more accurate than ^{18}F-FDG for glioma imaging. Another biologically similar amino acid imaging agent, ^{18}F-FET (^{18}F-fluoroethyl tyrosine), can also be used for the diagnosis of glioma, with high uptake indicating tumor cell proliferation. Recent studies have found that ^{18}F-FET may have a higher signal-to-noise ratio and lesion contrast. Neuroreceptor imaging agents, such as ^{18}F-FDOPA (^{18}F-dopamine), are increasingly being used for tumor imaging. ^{18}F-FDOPA is an exogenous neurotransmitter that regulates motor function, neural activity, and other physiological processes through dopamine receptors in the brain. Its high uptake is highly correlated with the tumor proliferation index Ki-67 and may even be used to differentiate HGG from LGG. Additionally, ^{18}F-FLT (^{18}F-fluorothymine) is a drug that reflects nucleotide metabolism, and its increased uptake represents increased cellular DNA synthesis, which can also aid in the diagnosis of gliomas. Compared to conventional MRI techniques, amino acid PET can improve the accuracy of outlining the biological boundary of tumors and detect potential infiltration/invasion of brain tissue by tumor cells that may not be detected on conventional MRI images. Therefore, PET combined with MRI can more accurately define the target area of radiotherapy than MRI alone.

7.7 Intraoperative MRI-Based Multimodal Image Navigation for Glioma Surgery

Maximizing safe resection of the glioma and preserving postoperative neurological status are essential prognostic factors for glioma surgery. Preoperative neuroimaging has evolved from basic structural imaging to functional and metabolic imaging, which enables more accurate delineation of tumor boundaries and their relationship to surrounding functional areas of the brain. Intraoperative MRI techniques have emerged due to the growing interest in preoperative image navigation. The development of intraoperative MRI technology from low to ultra-high field strength has enabled real-time imaging with high resolution, signal-to-noise ratio, and both structural and functional images. Preliminary results of our prospective randomized triple-blind controlled study show that intraoperative MRI increases the extent of glioma resection, particularly for LGG, and prolongs PFS in glioma patients. The combination of intraoperative MRI-based multimodal imaging with intraoperative resting-state functional imaging provides more information on the preservation of eloquent areas, allowing neurosurgeons to perform glioma resection more safely. Additionally, intraoperative MRI-based multimodal imaging can be combined with awake craniotomy, intraoperative electrophysiological techniques, and intraoperative fluorescein to improve the efficacy of glioma resection and prolong tumor-free survival while reducing the incidence of postoperative neurological deficits and improving quality of life.

Multimodal image navigation is also an important technique for biopsy surgeries when dealing with multifocal, diffuse, or deep-seated lesions. High Cho/NAA ratios on MRS images, high rCBV on PWI images, or high metabolic levels on PET images can be used as targets for biopsy. These targets are often located in densely tumor cell-populated areas with relatively high malignancy, improving the accuracy and efficiency of biopsy surgeries. Intraoperative MRI can also verify the accuracy of the target in real time, further improving the reliability of the biopsy results.

7.8 Artificial Intelligence (AI) Is Increasingly Being Utilized in the Diagnosis and Prediction of Glioma

Artificial intelligence is becoming increasingly important in the field of medical image analysis, providing effective solutions to a range of problems. The growing field of radiomics, which combines deep learning techniques with rapid image analysis, is poised to revolutionize radiological sciences. Deep learning, a subset of machine learning artificial intelligence, has shown promise in solving medical imaging-based problems. MRI is widely used to characterize gliomas, which are characterized by abnormal vascular proliferation, cell proliferation, tumor invasion, and apoptosis. However, labeling the different markers on MRI images can be difficult due to the heterogeneity of the tumors. Currently, deep learning is being used for pre- and post-operative tumor segmentation, genetic characterization of tissues, and prediction in the field of glioma diagnosis and outcome prediction. These deep learning methods are promising for research and development, enhancing scientific research and clinical practice by accurately diagnosing and treating gliomas.

It is important to note that, among the three elements of big data, strong computing power and precise algorithms can be continually improved through technological breakthroughs. However, ensuring the accuracy, reliability, and homogenization of big data during the process of accumulating quantity is crucial. This is the cornerstone for AI to play a powerful role in the field of glioma diagnosis and prediction.

Further Reading

Albert NL, Weller M, Suchorska B, et al. Response Assessment in Neuro-Oncology working group and European Association for Neuro-Oncology recommendations for the clinical use of PET imaging in gliomas. Neuro Oncol. 2016;18(9):1199–208.

Anbarloui MR, Ghodsi SM, Khoshnevisan A, et al. Accuracy of magnetic resonance spectroscopy in distinction between radiation necrosis and recurrence of brain tumors. Iran J Neurol. 2015;14(1):29–34.

Andronesi OC, Rapalino O, Gerstner E, et al. Detection of oncogenic IDH1 mutations using magnetic resonance spectroscopy of 2-hydroxyglutarate. J Clin Invest. 2013;123(9):3659–63.

Azadbakht H, Parkes LM, Haroon HA, et al. Validation of high-resolution tractography against in vivo tracing in the macaque visual cortex. Cereb Cortex. 2015;25(11):4299–309.

Barajas RF, Chang JS, Segal MR, et al. Differentiation of recurrent glioblastoma multiforme from radiation necrosis after external beam radiation therapy with dynamic susceptibility-weighted contrast-enhanced perfusion MR imaging. Radiology. 2009;253(2):486–96.

Bell C, Dowson N, Puttick S, et al. Increasing feasibility and utility of (18)F-FDOPA PET for the management of glioma. Nucl Med Biol. 2015;42(10):788–95.

Bello L, Castellano A, Fava E, et al. Intraoperative use of diffusion tensor imaging fiber tractography and subcortical mapping for resection of gliomas: technical considerations. Neurosurg Focus. 2010;28(2):E6.

Biswal B, Yetkin FZ, Haughton VM, et al. Functional connectivity in the motor cortex of resting human brain using echo-planar MRI. Magn Reson Med. 1995;34(4):537–41.

Brandão LA, Castillo M. Adult brain tumors: clinical applications of magnetic resonance spectroscopy. Neuroimaging Clin N Am. 2013;23(3):527–55.

Cha S, Lupo JM, Chen MH, et al. Differentiation of glioblastoma multiforme and single brain metastasis by peak height and percentage of signal intensity recovery derived from dynamic susceptibility-weighted contrast-enhanced perfusion MR imaging. AJNR Am J Neuroradiol. 2007;28(6):1078–84.

China Glioma Collaborative Group (CGCG). Guidelines for the surgical treatment of adult supratentorial low-grade gliomas. Chin J Neurosurg. 2016;32(7):652–8.

Choi C, Ganji SK, Deberardinis RJ, et al. 2-Hydroxyglutarate detection by magnetic resonance spectroscopy in IDH-mutated patients with gliomas. Nat Med. 2012;18(4):624–9.

De La Peña MJ, Robles SG, Rodríguez MR, et al. Cortical and subcortical mapping of language areas: correlation of functional MRI and tractography in a 3T scanner with intraoperative cortical and subcortical stimulation in patients with brain tumors located in eloquent areas. Radiologia. 2013;55(6):505–13.

Dunet V, Maeder P, Nicod-Lalonde M, et al. Combination of MRI and dynamic FET PET for initial glioma grading. Nuklearmedizin. 2014;53(4):155–61.

Dunet V, Pomoni A, Hottinger A, et al. Performance of 18F-FET versus 18F-FDG-PET for the diagnosis and grading of brain tumors: systematic review and meta-analysis. Neuro Oncol. 2016;18(3):426–34.

Farshidfar Z, Faeghi F, Mohseni M, et al. Diffusion tensor tractography in the presurgical assessment of cerebral gliomas. Neuroradiol J. 2014;27(1):75–84.

Ferdová E, Ferda J, Baxa J, et al. Assessment of grading in newly-diagnosed glioma using 18F-fluorothymidine PET/CT. Anticancer Res. 2015;35(2):955–9.

Fueger BJ, Czernin J, Cloughesy T, et al. Correlation of 6-18F-fluoro-L-dopa PET uptake with proliferation and tumor grade in newly diagnosed and recurrent gliomas. J Nucl Med. 2010;51(10):1532–8.

Götz I, Grosu AL. [(18)F]FET-PET imaging for treatment and response monitoring of radiation therapy in malignant glioma patients—a review. Front Oncol. 2013;3:104.

Guo J, Yao C, Chen H, et al. The relationship between Cho/NAA and glioma metabolism: implementation for margin delineation of cerebral gliomas. Acta Neurochir (Wien). 2012;154(8):1361–70.

Jack CR Jr, Thompson RM, Butts RK, et al. Sensory motor cortex: correlation of presurgical mapping with functional MR imaging and invasive cortical mapping. Radiology. 1994;190(1):85–92.

Kim SS, McCutcheon IE, Suki D, et al. Awake craniotomy for brain tumors near eloquent cortex: correlation of intraoperative cortical mapping with neurological outcomes in consecutive 309 patients. Neurosurgery. 2009;64(5):836–45.

Kobayashi K, Hirata K, Yamaguchi S, et al. Prognostic value of volume-based measurements on (11) C-methionine PET in glioma patients. Eur J Nucl Med Mol Imaging. 2015;42(7):1071–80.

Kokkonen SM, Nikkinen J, Remes J, et al. Preoperative localization of the sensorimotor area using independent component analysis of resting-state fMRI. Magn Reson Imaging. 2009;27(6):733–40.

Lau EW, Drummond KJ, Ware RE, et al. Comparative PET study using F-18 FET and F-18 FDG for the evaluation of patients with suspected brain tumour. J Clin Neurosci. 2010;17(1):43–9.

Leclercq D, Duffau H, Delmaire C, et al. Comparison of diffusion tensor imaging tractography of language tracts and intraoperative subcortical stimulations. J Neurosurg. 2010;112(3):503–11.

Liang D, Schulder M. The role of intraoperative magnetic resonance imaging in glioma surgery. Surg Neurol Int. 2012;3(Suppl 4):S320–7.

Liang R, Wang X, Li M, et al. Meta-analysis of peritumoural rCBV values derived from dynamic susceptibility contrast imaging in differentiating high-grade gliomas from intracranial metastases. Int J Clin Exp Med. 2014a;7(9):2724–9.

Liang R, Li M, Wang X, et al. Role of rCBV values derived from dynamic susceptibility contrast-enhanced magnetic resonance imaging in differentiating CNS lymphoma from high grade glioma: a meta-analysis. Int J Clin Exp Med. 2014b;7(12a):5573–7.

Liu H, Buckner RL, Talukdar T, et al. Task-free presurgical mapping using functional magnetic resonance imaging intrinsic activity. J Neurosurg. 2009;111(4): 746–54.

Lotumolo A, Caivano R, Rabasco P, et al. Comparison between magnetic resonance spectroscopy and diffusion weighted imaging in the evaluation of gliomas response after treatment. Eur J Radiol. 2015;84(12):2597–604.

Lu J, Wu J, Yao C, et al. Awake language mapping and 3-Tesla intraoperative MRI-guided volumetric resection for gliomas in language areas. J Clin Neurosci. 2013;20(9):1280–7.

National Health Care Commission Medical Administration. Glioma diagnosis and treatment standard (annual 2018 edition). Chin J Neurosurg. 2019;35(3):217–39.

Nihashi T, Dahabreh IJ, Terasawa T. PET in the clinical management of glioma: evidence map. AJR Am J Roentgenol. 2013;200(6):W654–60.

Pujol S, Wells W, Pierpaoli C, et al. The DTI challenge: towards standardized evaluation of diffusion tensor imaging tractography for neurosurgery. J Neuroimaging. 2015;25(5):875–82.

Puttick S, Bell C, Dowson N, et al. PET, MRI, and simultaneous PET/MRI in the development of diagnostic and therapeutic strategies for glioma. Drug Discov Today. 2015;20(3):306–17.

Qiu TM, Zhang Y, Wu JS, et al. Virtual reality presurgical planning for cerebral gliomas adjacent to motor pathways in an integrated 3-D stereoscopic visualization of structural MRI and DTI tractography. Acta Neurochir (Wien). 2010;152(11):1847–57.

Qiu TM, Yao CJ, Wu JS, et al. Clinical experience of 3T intraoperative magnetic resonance imaging integrated neurosurgical suite in Shanghai Huashan Hospital. Chin Med J (Engl). 2012;125(24):4328–33.

Qiu TM, Yan CG, Tang WJ, et al. Localizing hand motor area using resting-state fMRI: validated with direct cortical stimulation. Acta Neurochir (Wien). 2014;156(12):2295–302.

Qiu TM, Gong FY, Gong X, et al. Real-time motor cortex mapping for the safe resection of glioma: an Intraoperative resting-state fMRI study. AJNR Am J Neuroradiol. 2017;38(11):2146–52.

Raichle ME. A brief history of human brain mapping. Trends Neurosci. 2009;32(2):118–26.

Raichle ME. Two views of brain function. Trends Cogn Sci. 2010;14(4):180–90.

Raichle ME. The restless brain. Brain Connect. 2011;1(1):3–12.

Sanai N, Berger MS. Intraoperative stimulation techniques for functional pathway preservation and glioma resection. Neurosurg Focus. 2010;28(2):E1.

Shaver MM, Kohanteb PA, Chiou C, et al. Optimizing neuro-oncology imaging: a review of deep learning approaches for glioma imaging. Cancers (Basel). 2019;11(6):829.

Shields AF, Grierson JR, Dohmen BM, et al. Imaging proliferation in vivo with [F-18]FLT and positron emission tomography. Nat Med. 1998;4(11):1334–6.

Shimony JS, Zhang D, Johnston JM, et al. Resting-state spontaneous fluctuations in brain activity: a new paradigm for presurgical planning using fMRI. Acad Radiol. 2009;16(5):578–83.

Specialized Committee on Glioma, Neurosurgeons Branch, Chinese Medical Association. Multidisciplinary diagnosis and treatment of glioma (MDT) Chinese Expert Consensus. Chin J Neurosurg. 2018;34(2):113–8.

Tang C, Guo J, Chen H, et al. Gene mutation profiling of primary glioblastoma through multiple tumor biopsy guided by 1H-magnetic resonance spectroscopy. Int J Clin Exp Pathol. 2015;8(5):5327–35.

Tie Y, Rigolo L, Norton IH, et al. Defining language networks from resting-state fMRI for surgical planning—a feasibility study. Hum Brain Mapp. 2014;35(3):1018–30.

Tong T, Yang Z, Chen JW, et al. Dynamic 1H-MRS assessment of brain tumors: a novel approach for differential diagnosis of glioma. Oncotarget. 2015;6(31):32257–65.

Villani V, Carapella CM, Chiaravalloti A, et al. The role of PET [18F]FDOPA in evaluating low-grade glioma. Anticancer Res. 2015;35(9):5117–22.

Weller M, van den Bent M, Hopkins K, et al. EANO guideline for the diagnosis and treatment of anaplastic gliomas and glioblastoma. Lancet Oncol. 2014;15(9):e395–403.

Wu JS, Zhang J, Zhuang DX, et al. Current status of cerebral glioma surgery in China. Chin Med J (Engl). 2011;124(17):2569–77.

Wu JS, Gong X, Song YY, et al. 3.0-T intraoperative magnetic resonance imaging-guided resection in cerebral glioma surgery: interim analysis of a prospective, randomized, triple-blind, parallel-controlled trial. Neurosurgery. 2014;61(Suppl 1):145–54.

Xing Z, You RX, Li J, et al. Differentiation of primary central nervous system lymphomas from high-grade gliomas by rCBV and percentage of signal intensity recovery derived from dynamic susceptibility-weighted contrast-enhanced perfusion MR imaging. Clin Neuroradiol. 2014;24(4):329–36.

Yetkin FZ, Mueller WM, Morris GL, et al. Functional MR activation correlated with intraoperative cortical mapping. AJNR Am J Neuroradiol. 1997;18(7): 1311–5.

Yoon JH, Kim JH, Kang WJ, et al. Grading of cerebral glioma with multiparametric MR imaging and18 F-FDG-PET: concordance and accuracy. Eur Radiol. 2014;24(2):380–9.

Zhang D, Raichle ME. Disease and the brain's dark energy. Nat Rev Neurol. 2010;6(1):15–28.

Zhang D, Johnston JM, Fox MD, et al. Preoperative sensorimotor mapping in brain tumor patients using spontaneous fluctuations in neuronal activity imaged with functional magnetic resonance imaging: initial experience. Neurosurgery. 2009;65(6 Suppl):226–36.

Zhang Y, Wan SH, Wu GJ, et al. Magnetic resonance diffusion tensor imaging and diffusion tensor tractography of the human visual pathway. Int J Ophthalmol. 2012;5(4):452–8.

Zhu FP, Wu JS, Song YY, et al. Clinical application of motor pathway mapping using diffusion tensor imaging tractography and intraoperative direct subcortical stimulation in cerebral glioma surgery: a prospective cohort study. Neurosurgery. 2012;71(6): 1170–83.

Brain Function Studies in the Perioperative Period of Glioma

8

Liang Chen

8.1 Understanding the History of Brain Function Research Has Important Practical Implications

Despite the significant progress made in understanding the brain through modern scientific research, there is still much more to be discovered. Before delving deeper into this field, it is crucial to understand the history of brain function research. By examining the methods and techniques that have been used to unlock the secrets of the brain over time, we can gain a better appreciation for the scientific process and technical approach that has led to current understanding. This section provides a chronological overview of the most significant historical events in brain function research, allowing us to build a foundation for further exploration and understanding of this complex field.

The history of the objective exploration of brain function spans over 200 years. Prior to this, theories such as the "gas theory" of the second century AD and the "ventricle theory" of the late fourth century AD were based on subjective inferences and lacked anatomical and structural bases. The first scholar to use detailed anatomical knowledge to revise the ventricle theory, which had dominated academic thought for over a millennium, was Andreas Vesalius. In 1543, he published an anatomical treatise detailing the structure of the brain, which spurred subsequent scholars to explore brain function in relation to brain structure. By the early eighteenth century, the anatomist Franz Joseph Gall and his student Johann Gaspar Spurzheim proposed the existence of cortical regions in the brain responsible for different functions. Their six-volume *Anatomy and Physiology of the Nervous System* laid the groundwork for the study of brain function based on brain structure. Although their ideas were not immediately embraced by the scientific community, their work contributed to the understanding and study of brain function. Today, these early studies remain of great scientific significance, providing the theoretical basis and research methods for all future scientists studying brain function.

In the nineteenth century, with the invention of the microscope, the establishment of the cell theory, and the maturation of brain anatomy, the study of brain function developed rapidly. The relationship between the brain and human mental cognition was more accurately described than Luigi Rolando by Flaurens Pierre, who used animal experiments to remove different brain structures and observe the function of each part of the brain. He believed that brain functions are all isotropic and that the brain works as a unified whole, and he pioneered the use of animal experiments to study the functions of different brain struc-

L. Chen (✉)
Department of Neurosurgery, Huashan Hospital, Fudan University, Shanghai, China
e-mail: hschenliang@fudan.edu.cn

Y. Mao (ed.), *Progress in the Diagnosis and Treatment of Gliomas*, Experts' Perspectives on Medical Advances, https://doi.org/10.1007/978-981-99-0123-4_8

tures, becoming the founder of brain physiology. The careful observation of patients by clinicians also led to breakthroughs in the functional study of the human brain. In 1861, the French neurologist P. Broca found that a patient with aphasia was associated with a lesion in the posterior left frontal lobe, linking the loss of oral speech to a localized brain injury, and the brain region was named Broca's area, a motor speech cortex.

In 1874, Wernicke observed a patient with a lesion in the posterior left superior temporal gyrus who could pronounce words correctly but spoke incoherently and had impaired comprehension of language. This brain region was named Wernicke's area, a sensory language cortex. Almost simultaneously, German psychiatrists Gustav Fritsch and Eduard Hitzig electrically stimulated different areas of the anterior part of the Daquan hemisphere to obtain contractile movements of the contralateral body muscles, finding five different motor points. However, they did not stimulate the posterior part of the hemisphere to obtain muscle movements, thus confirming the existence of separate motor centers in the brain. David Ferrier, a British neurologist, later replicated the results of Fritsch and Hitzig's electrical stimulation experiments on monkey and dog brains, establishing the principle of localization of sensory and motor functions in the brain. Roberts Bartholow, an American neurosurgeon, was the first person to perform electrical stimulation on the human brain. In 1874, he conducted a trial of electrical stimulation on the cerebral cortex of a patient with an ulcerated skull and exposed meninges. He described in detail how stimulation with weak currents in some cortical areas caused contraction of some muscles, while stimulation in other cortical areas was accompanied by subjective sensation. Strong currents resulted in foaming at the mouth and limb spasms.

In the twentieth century, both Harvey Cushing of the United States and the Canadian neurologist W. G. Penfield made significant contributions to the precise localization of brain function through extensive electrical stimulation of the human brain. Penfield's homunculus, which accurately depicts the distribution of motor, sensory, and visual cortices in the brain, remains a classic model. Penfield used direct cortical stimulation (DCS) during arousal surgery under local anesthesia of the scalp. The observation of patients with brain injuries during the two world wars of the twentieth century also provided a wealth of information for studying the human brain. These approaches, either directly or indirectly invasive, are relatively intuitive and convincing. With the development of science and technology in the twentieth century, noninvasive methods for observing brain structure and function became possible. The invention of electroencephalography (EEG) in the late 1920s and its development in the 1960s, along with the invention of event-related potential (ERP) and magnetoencephalography (MEG), allowed for real-time recording of EEG changes during events related to brain function. The development of MEG has also enabled real-time recording of EEG changes during events related to brain function. The invention of PET, functional magnetic resonance imaging (fMRI), and functional near-infrared spectroscopy (fNIRS) has enabled physicians to observe and measure the brain's blood flow, function, and activity during the performance of specific tasks. In the twenty-first century, the rapid development of neurobiology techniques such as single cell recording, multi-cell recording, array electrode recording, and histochemical neurotransmitter measurement has enabled scientists to study brain function at the cellular and molecular levels.

This review of the history of brain function research can enhance our ability to apply brain function research to clinical practice and advance brain science exploration.

8.2 Complementary Technologies for Better Clinical Application of Functional Brain Imaging in Glioma

Accurate preoperative and intraoperative functional brain localization is critical in glioma surgery to preserve neurological function and reduce postoperative disability rates. Different techniques for functional brain localization have their respective advantages and disadvantages, making it important to investigate how they can be applied accurately for individualized surgery. This section provides an overview of two broad categories of functional brain imaging techniques: electrophysiological and metabolic imaging. Electrophysiological techniques, including EEG, MEG, TMS, and DCS, directly measure neuroelectrical activity, while PET, SPECT, fMRI, and fNIRS are indirect measurement techniques that reflect local compound metabolism in the brain. Table 8.1 summarizes the characteristics of these techniques in brain function localization. Currently, a combination of both types of techniques is used in perioperative brain function localization for glioma surgery, applied on a case-by-case basis to achieve precise brain function localization and protection.

Table 8.1 Characteristics of brain function localization techniques

	Electrophysiological techniques (direct)				Local metabolism or blood oxygen imaging technology in the brain (indirect)			
	EEG	MEG	TMS	DCS	PET	SPECT	fMRI	fNIRS
Disadvantage	Need to wear an electrode cap, low spatial resolution, unable to explore deep neural activity in the brain	Expensive price, high requirements for environmental shielding, low spatial resolution, only able to detect shallow cerebral cortex	Strict parameters such as spike frequency need to be set, but there are still certain safety issues	It needs to be completed after craniotomy, and the incidence of epilepsy is high, so whole brain testing cannot be performed	Expensive price, requires intravenous injection of isotopic contrast agents, cannot perform multimodal brain imaging	Intravenous injection of isotope contrast agent is required, and isotope decay is slow, making it impossible to perform multimodal brain imaging	The time resolution is slightly low, only sensitive to deoxyhemoglobin, and greatly affected by magnetic field environment and coils	Can only reflect superficial cerebral cortex, low spatial resolution, requires wearing an infrared probe cap
Advantage	Directly reflecting neural electrical activity, cocoa can be detected for a long time, inexpensive, and movable	Directly reflecting neural electrical activity, with high temporal resolution, and no contact between the detector and the scalp	Directly reflecting neural electrical activity, capable of deep stimulation, and can itself be used as a treatment method	Direct real-time reflection of cortical function, which can be used for superficial and deep stimulation	Low dosage of radioactive reagents, high image contrast, and fast decay rate of radioactive isotopes	The half-life of radioactive isotopes is longer, the dosage is smaller, and the detection process is relatively simple	No radiation damage, high spatial resolution, capable of performing multimodal brain imaging	Simultaneously reflecting the content of deoxyhemoglobin and oxygenated hemoglobin, it can detect multiple people simultaneously, and the testing time can be longer

8.3 Multimodal Functional Imaging Is the Predominant Method for Preoperative Functional Brain Localization

Various preoperative functional brain localization techniques are available for glioma, including multimodal functional imaging, EEG, MEG, and PET. Multimodal functional imaging is currently the most commonly used technique in clinical practice. Advances in functional imaging techniques have enabled preoperative brain functional localization to progress from two-dimensional imaging to three-dimensional reproduction, from structural and functional separation to fusion, from localization of primary brain functions to higher cognitive functions, and from task-based to resting-state functional imaging. Multimodal functional imaging encompasses conventional structural imaging, fiber tract tracer imaging based on DTI technology, and task-based and resting-state BOLD imaging based on blood oxygen levels.

Conventional structural imaging is the primary preoperative tool used to determine the relationship between glioma and functional areas. It provides information about cerebral sulci and gyri, the preliminary determination of tumor growth pattern, the extent of invasion, and functional areas associated with the tumor, helping to choose more accurate functional brain localization techniques. In the preoperative period, a careful review of conventional imaging findings should be combined with a detailed neurological examination of the patient's clinical presentation. This includes a thorough inquiry about preoperative symptoms and their course and understanding the location of epilepsy aura to assess preoperative neurological status. This evaluation is particularly important in the perioperative assessment of temporal lobe gliomas. The following is a case of a preoperative Wada test and cognitive function assessment.

Case The patient was admitted to the hospital with "recurrent right hemifacial hot flashes," and a cranial MRI revealed diffuse LGG in the left frontotemporal lobe. Consequently, a Wada test and cognitive function assessment were conducted before surgery to identify the functional lateralization of the patient's brain. Results showed that the left side of the brain was primarily responsible for memory and language, and the patient had normal cognitive function. During surgery, the tumor lesion was completely excised from the right hippocampus. After surgery, the patient's memory, language, and cognitive functions remained normal, as seen in Fig. 8.1.

DTI-based fiber bundle tracer imaging is a valuable technique for localizing subcortical fiber bundles. It enables neurosurgeons to understand the spatial anatomical relationship between lesions and fiber bundles, formulate preoperative plans, and guide the scope and direction of subcortical electrical stimulation during surgery. In a previous randomized controlled study, we found that the use of DTI navigation technology reduced the incidence of motor dysfunction after glioma surgery by minimizing medical injury to the pyramidal fasciculus. Imaging of the arcuate fibers also helped reduce the occurrence of postoperative language dysfunction. However, it is important to note that DTI tracer imaging has many variables, and the imaging results are often highly uncertain. Future research should focus on distinguishing different functional fiber bundles, assessing the actual travel and function of fiber bundles deformed by lesion compression, and accurately setting tracer parameters.

Task-based and resting-state BOLD imaging are commonly used techniques for preoperative functional brain localization in glioma surgery. Traditional BOLD techniques are task-based, and preoperative motor BOLD and speech BOLD are routine functional imaging examinations before tumor resection in functional areas. Motor BOLD is more accurate in localizing motor areas, while speech BOLD is slightly less sensitive and specific in visualizing speech areas. Recently, resting-state BOLD imaging has also been applied to functional brain localization in glioma surgery, providing complementary information to task-based imaging. However, it is important to note that BOLD imaging is statistically based and may lead to false positives and false negatives, which neurosurgeons should be aware of during interpretation.

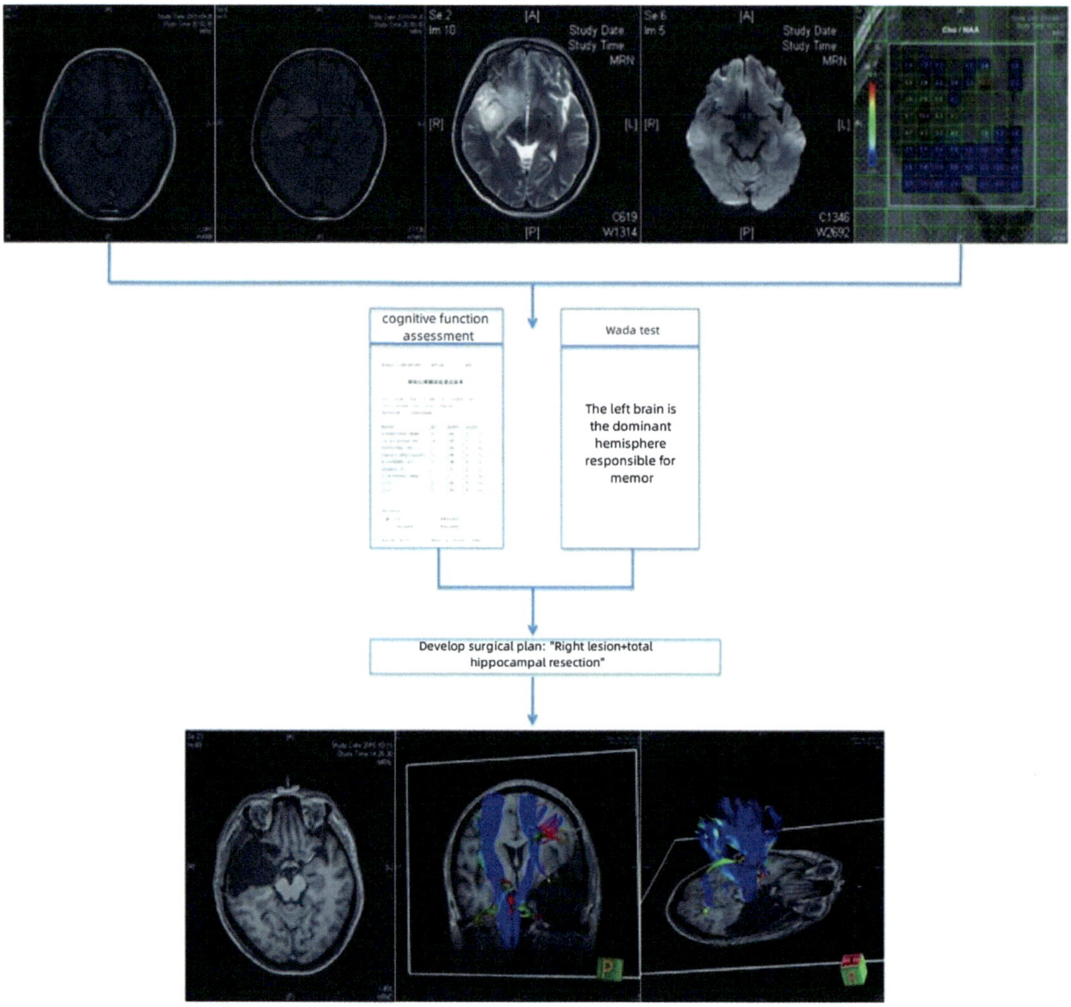

Fig. 8.1 Application of Wada trial and cognitive function assessment in clinical cases

Multimodal imaging involves the integration of conventional structural images, DTI images depicting conduction tracts, and BOLD images highlighting functional cortex to generate a three-dimensional image. While imaging is an indirect technique and cannot replace electrophysiological techniques as it does not represent actual neuronal electrical activity, it holds significant clinical value in preoperatively assessing the spatial anatomy of the lesion in relation to functional cortical and subcortical conduction tracts. This helps the neurosurgeon plan preoperatively, identify important functional areas that may be approached intraoperatively, reduce unnecessary electrical stimulation, and minimize the incidence of seizures due to electrical stimulation, thereby reducing the likelihood of epilepsy.

8.4 Electrophysiological Techniques Remain the Most Reliable Standard for Intraoperative Brain Function Localization

The history of brain function research shows that electrophysiological techniques have played a crucial role in localizing brain function from the beginning, and most of the current concepts and knowledge of functional brain cortex are derived from electrophysiological techniques. With the standardization and popularization of electrophysiological techniques, it has become a routine technique for functional localization and monitoring in functional glioma surgery and is currently the most reliable standard for intraoperative brain functional localization. Somatosensory evoked potential (SEP) can be used to determine the central sulcus by inverting the evoked potential, which is also a method to monitor the function of spinal cord segments and spinal nerves during spinal cord glioma resection. Motor evoked potential (MEP) can be used for intraoperative motor area localization and monitoring motor pathways during tumor resection. Direct cortical electrical stimulation can be used for intraoperative localization of motor and speech cortices, while direct subcortical electrical stimulation can be used to localize motor and speech pathways. However, when using intraoperative electrophysiological techniques for localization and monitoring of brain function, attention should be paid to the following factors: (1) preparation for possible seizures, including the use of anesthetic drugs and ice saline rinsing, proper fixation of the head frame, and keeping away from the cortex during subcortical electrical stimulation; (2) close cooperation with anesthesia, including the use of sedatives and muscle relaxants, to ensure accurate reference values for electrophysiological results; (3) the use of arousal anesthesia for language cortical localization (the maturity of arousal anesthesia techniques is a guarantee of safety); (4) electrophysiological techniques are not completely accurate, and there may be delays in the monitoring process, which require accurate interpretation and judgment of electrophysiological results; and (5) effective combination of anatomical and functional imaging information will help improve the efficiency of electrophysiological localization of functional brain areas and reduce the occurrence of adverse events such as epilepsy.

In recent years, the use of intraoperative MRI has enabled the collection and application of real-time functional imaging data during surgery. Intraoperative task-state MRI and resting-state functional MRI under general anesthesia can provide real-time functional area information and reduce errors caused by brain displacement. The use of intraoperative corticocortical-cortical electrophysiological monitoring techniques can assist neurosurgeons in the localization and scientific study of cortical and subcortical functional networks. In addition, intraoperative real-time cortical EEG recording and deep electrode placement video, as well as long-range EEG monitoring, are not only important monitoring techniques for tumor surgery related to epilepsy but also important technical tools for brain function research.

8.5 Online Real-Time Brain Function Localization

The current methods for localizing neurocortical function, particularly the motor area, include microsurgery, neuroimaging, and neurophysiological techniques. However, these methods have limitations that impact their ability to meet the needs of functional brain surgery in terms of speed, accuracy, and safety. Neuroimaging techniques, such as fMRI and PET, have limitations in their ability to monitor the surgical process and determine the functional status of the brain in real-time. fMRI has an error rate of 5–10 mm, while PET has a compliance rate of only 65% with electrophysiological stimulation. Neurophysiological techniques, such as direct cortical or subcortical stimulation, have an intraoperative accuracy of 5 mm. However, these techniques are limited by the potential risk of damage to the cerebral cortex and triggering epilepsy, as well as being a cumbersome process. Therefore, current functional brain localization methods are not able to fully meet the needs of surgery in functional brain areas, specifically in terms of speed, accuracy, and safety.

Electrode cortical graph (ECoG) has recently gained significant attention as a functional brain localization technique due to its numerous advantages. Firstly, ECoG localizes brain functions through passive detection, without the need for electrical stimulation, thereby avoiding potential risks associated with the stimulation process. Secondly, electrical stimulation requires time-consuming point-by-point cortical stimulation, which limits localization to a small area around the stimulation point. In contrast, ECoG can rapidly achieve functional localization across a broader area of the brain. Furthermore, signal analysis can be used to obtain functional correlations between different brain areas, enabling more comprehensive evaluation and localization of functional areas. Thirdly, ECoG functional localization requires less patient cooperation compared to electrocortical stimulation, which is challenging for patients with cognitive dysfunction, children, and the elderly. Lastly, ECoG can be used to determine functional areas initially, followed by cortical stimulation to precisely locate them, thus reducing the range of cortical stimulation trials in cases where it is necessary.

During arousal anesthesia, cortical electrodes are applied after the dura mater is cut, and a resting EEG is collected as a baseline. Recent advancements in algorithm optimization and cortical electrode hardware technology have made it possible to localize electrode sites online in real time using BCI2000 and SIGFRIED algorithms. These algorithms show the functional correlation of each electrode site with the current paradigm, allowing for intraoperative preservation. The main advantage of this technique is that the relationship between the discharge area and the functional paradigm can be analyzed based on the brain's natural firing characteristics without the need for electrical stimulation. However, the algorithm is still in its early stages, and its accuracy requires further testing. Despite this, it is expected that this technique will soon replace cortical electrical stimulation as the new standard for functional brain localization.

With the establishment of brain programs around the world and the launch of the Brain Functional Connectivity Group, the concept of brain networks has been introduced, raising questions about how we locate brain function. Is there a one-to-one correspondence between the cerebral cortex and brain function, or do brain networks work together to achieve brain functions? What are the structural, anatomical, cellular, and molecular mechanisms by which these brain networks achieve brain function? How does brain function change prior to and after tumor resection, and what kind of remodeling occurs? Additionally, when we use ERP and fMRI to localize brain function, we must consider whether the task design is reasonable and how to improve spatial and temporal resolution. Finally, what are the unique properties of functional brain connections beyond connection strength and projection direction?

The answers to these questions require the development of technologies with higher spatial and temporal resolution that can complement and integrate various technologies, not only for brain science research but also for clinical applications. Neurosurgeons have the advantage of utilizing various technologies to work directly with the human brain, and the challenge of exploring and protecting the brain is a constant one.

Further Reading

De Witt Hamer PC, Robles SG, Zwinderman AH, et al. Impact of intraoperative stimulation brain mapping on glioma surgery outcome: a meta-analysis. J Clin Oncol. 2012;30(20):2559–65.

Diekhoff S, Uludağ K, Sparing R, et al. Functional localization in the human brain: gradient-echo, spin-echo, and arterial spin-labeling fMRI compared with neuronavigated TMS. Hum Brain Mapp. 2011;32(3):341–57.

Farshidfar Z, Faeghi F, Mohseni M, et al. Diffusion tensor tractography in the presurgical assessment of cerebral gliomas. Neuroradiol J. 2014;27(1):75–84.

Gallagher A, Beland R, Lassonde M. The contribution of functional near-infrared spectroscopy (fNIRS) to the presurgical assessment of language function in children. Brain Lang. 2012;121(2):124–9.

Lu J, Wu J, Yao C, et al. Awake language mapping and 3-Tesla intraoperative MRI-guided volumetric resection for gliomas in language areas. J Clin Neurosci. 2013;20(9):1280–7.

Maesawa S, Fujii M, Nakahara N, et al. Intraoperative tractography and motor evoked potential (MEP) monitoring in surgery for gliomas around the corticospinal tract. World Neurosurg. 2010;74(1):153–61.

Mormina E, Longo M, Arrigo A, et al. MRI tractography of corticospinal tract and arcuate fasciculus in high-grade gliomas performed by constrained spherical deconvolution: qualitative and quantitative analysis. Am J Neuroradiol. 2015;36(10):1853–8.

Nihashi T, Dahabreh IJ, Terasawa T. PET in the clinical management of glioma: evidence map. AJR Am J Roentgenol. 2013;200(6):W654–60.

Pujol S, Wells W, Pierpaoli C, et al. The DTI challenge: towards standardized evaluation of diffusion tensor imaging tractography for neurosurgery. J Neuroimaging. 2015;25(6):875–82.

Qiu TM, Zhang Y, Wu JS, et al. Virtual reality presurgical planning for cerebral gliomas adjacent to motor pathways in an integrated 3-D stereoscopic visualization of structural MRI and DTI tractography. Acta Neurochir (Wien). 2010;15(11):1847–57.

Qiu TM, Yao CJ, Wu JS, et al. Clinical experience of 3T intraoperative magnetic resonance imaging integrated neurosurgical suite in Shanghai Huashan Hospital. Chin Med J (Engl). 2012;125(24):4328–33.

Qiu TM, Yan CG, Tang WJ, et al. Localizing hand motor area using resting-state fMRI: validated with direct cortical stimulation. Acta Neurochir (Wien). 2014;156(12):2295–302.

Tsuzuki D, Dan I. Spatial registration for functional near-infrared spectroscopy: from channel position on the scalp to cortical location in individual and group analyses. Neuroimage. 2014;85(Pt 1):92–103.

Vassal F, Schneider F, Nuti C. Intraoperative use of diffusion tensor imaging-based tractography for resection of gliomas located near the pyramidal tract: comparison with subcortical stimulation mapping and contribution to surgical outcomes. Br J Neurosurg. 2013;27(5):668–75.

Wu JS, Zhang J, Zhuang DX, et al. Current status of cerebral glioma surgery in China. Chin Med J (Engl). 2011;124(17):2569–77.

Wu JS, Gong X, Song YY, et al. 3.0-T intraoperative magnetic resonance imaging-guided resection in cerebral glioma surgery: interim analysis of a prospective, randomized, triple-blind, parallel-controlled trial. Neurosurgery. 2014;61(Suppl 1):145–54.

Yau JM, Hua J, Liao DA, et al. Efficient and robust identification of cortical targets in concurrent TMS–fMRI experiments. Neuroimage. 2013;76(1):134–44.

Zhang Y, Wan SH, Wu GJ, et al. Magnetic resonance diffusion tensor imaging and diffusion tensor tractography of the human visual pathway. Int J Ophthalmol. 2012;5(4):452–8.

Zhu FP, Wu JS, Song YY, et al. Clinical application of motor pathway mapping using diffusion tensor imaging tractography and intraoperative direct subcortical stimulation in cerebral glioma surgery: a prospective cohort study. Neurosurgery. 2012;71(6):1170–83.

9 Molecular Biomarker-Based Chemotherapy and Targeted Therapy for Glioma

Xin Zhang, Yu Yao, and Nan Zhou

9.1 Current Research Advances in Chemotherapy Regimens for Glioma

Gliomas encompass several histotypes, including pilocytic astrocytoma, astrocytoma, oligodendroglioma, and GBM. In recent years, numerous genomic studies of brain tumors have identified various genetic alterations and signaling pathways associated with glioma. Specifically, BRAF mutations/fusions in pilocytic astrocytomas, IDH1 mutations and 1p/19q co-deletions in oligodendrogliomas, and IDH mutations in gliomas with different prognosis have been identified. IDH mutations divide gliomas into two groups with distinct prognosis: the group with IDH mutation has a better prognosis, while the group with IDH wild type has a poor prognosis. LGG or GBM patients with IDH wild type often have EGFR amplification and PTEN deletion. Additionally, MGMT methylation is a predictive marker for the efficacy of TMZ chemotherapy in GBM patients. The TCGA study revealed that GBM can be classified into proneuronal, neuronal, classic, and mesenchymal subtypes based on mRNA expression and DNA methylation profiles. The inclusion of molecular pathology such as IDH and 1p/19q co-deletion in the WHO's 2016 classification of CNS malignant tumors is a significant advance in the study of molecular pathology of gliomas. Nonetheless, the average survival of gliomas, particularly HGG, remains brief.

Chemotherapy is commonly used to treat patients with low-grade gliomas (LGG), with temozolomide, procarbazine, ACNU, lomustine, and vincristine being the most frequently used regimen. The RTOG 9802 clinical trial demonstrated that combining radiotherapy with the PCV regimen (procarbazine, lomustine, and vincristine) provides survival benefits for patients with high-risk LGG. However, due to the lack of a direct comparison between the two regimens, some physicians still prefer oral temozolomide therapy as it is more convenient to administer. There is also no consensus on when to start chemotherapy after LGG surgery, the duration of chemotherapy, or whether to combine it with radiotherapy. Clinical research on molecular markers has made significant progress, with retrospective studies indicating that IDH mutations may predict the sensitivity of glioma patients to adjuvant therapies such as radiotherapy and chemotherapy. The long-term follow-up results of clinical trial RTOG 9402 showed that the sensitivity of the PCV regimen for anaplastic oligodendrogliomas was significantly correlated with IDH mutation. Therefore, glioma patients with IDH mutations have a better prognosis and are

X. Zhang · Y. Yao · N. Zhou (✉)
Department of Neurosurgery, Huashan Hospital, Fudan University, Shanghai, China

Y. Mao (ed.), *Progress in the Diagnosis and Treatment of Gliomas*, Experts' Perspectives on Medical Advances, https://doi.org/10.1007/978-981-99-0123-4_9

more sensitive to adjuvant therapy than those with IDH wild type.

In 2005, Stupp introduced the regimen of concurrent radiotherapy and TMZ chemotherapy, which has extended the average survival of GBM patients from 12.1 to 14.6 months and increased the 2-year survival rate from 12.1 to 26.5%. Although this represents a significant advance in glioma treatment, there is still a considerable scope for improvement. As a result, neurosurgeons and neuro-oncologists are pursuing targeted therapies based on gene mutations or molecular markers associated with the biological behavior of gliomas. This has become a crucial goal of research in the field.

The current standard treatment for newly diagnosed GBM involves the maximum safe resection of the tumor, followed by concurrent radiotherapy/TMZ chemotherapy and six courses of TMZ-adjuvant chemotherapy. Despite this approach, some studies have sought to overcome resistance to TMZ by modifying the dosing regimen. However, the RTOG0525 clinical trial found no significant difference in progression-free survival (PFS) and overall survival (OS) between patients with newly diagnosed GBM who were administered TMZ using either 21/28 consecutive low-dose regimens (75–100 mg/m^2) after concurrent radiotherapy, or conventional TMZ for 5/28 days. Nevertheless, both groups showed a prognostic predictive effect of MGMT methylation, suggesting longer OS. The GEINO 14-01 clinical trial also demonstrated that extending the duration of TMZ adjuvant therapy did not increase OS in GBM, while the RTOG0825 and AVAglio trials showed that adding targeted agents at the time of initial presentation did not prolong OS in GBM patients either.

Currently, there is no consensus on the standard treatment for recurrent gliomas. In some cases, redo surgery or second radiotherapy may be appropriate, depending on the individual circumstances. However, more frequently, chemotherapy or alternative treatments such as tumor treating fields (TTF) are used. Chemotherapy after relapse typically involves the use of alkylating agents such as lomustine, but patients with unmethylated MGMT promoters often do not respond well to these drugs. Furthermore, there have been fewer reports in recent years of continuing temozolomide treatment after tumor recurrence.

9.2 Molecular Subtypes of Gliomas and Chemotherapy

In 2016, the World Health Organization (WHO) revised the classification of central nervous system (CNS) tumors to include molecular genetic biomarkers for complete classification of adult diffuse gliomas. These biomarkers include IDH1/IDH2 mutation and 1p/19q co-deletion. Additionally, the TERT promoter is emerging as a crucial molecular marker for gliomas, which has prognostic value when used in combination with IDH1/IDH2 mutation and 1p/19q status.

The Cancer Genome Atlas (TCGA) performed a high-throughput somatic cell assay on glioblastoma multiforme (GBM) and lower-grade gliomas (WHO grade II–III), which classified glioma into three subtypes: IDH-mutant and 1p/19q co-deleted, IDH-mutant and non-co-deleted, and IDH wild type. Further research by Eckel-Passow showed that the combination of IDH, 1p/19q co-deletion, and TERT promoter can classify gliomas into five subgroups with different prognostic and mutation features. It is possible that different subgroups of glioma patients would have varying sensitivities to a single adjuvant treatment modality.

A 2014 article by Hai Yan's team at Duke University demonstrated that malignant gliomas could be classified into four subtypes based on IDH and TERTp mutation: IDH mut/TERTpmut, IDHmut/TERTwt, IDHwt/TERTpmut, and IDHwt/TERTpwt. The prognosis of these subtypes was significantly different, with IDHmut/TERTpmut having the best prognosis, followed by IDHmut/TERTpwt, IDHwt/TERTpwt, and IDHwt/TERTpmut having the worst prognosis. This classification method is simpler and more practical than the TCGA typing based on high-throughput sequencing.

The study aimed to investigate the relationship between IDH1/IDH2 expression, TERTp mutation, and overall survival (OS) in 473 adult glioma patients. The results showed that TERTp mutation was present in 74.2% of glioblastoma multiforme (GBM) patients but only in 18.2% of grade II–III astrocytoma patients. Conversely, IDH1/IDH2 mutation was prevalent in 78.4% of grade II–III astrocytoma patients, but uncommon in primary GBM. In oligodendrogliomas, the coexistence of TERTp and IDH1/IDH2 mutations was present in 79% of cases.

The survival analysis indicated that patients with IDH wild-type and TERTp mutations had the worst prognosis, with a median OS of 11.5 months, primarily due to primary GBM. Patients with IDH1/IDH2 mutation and TERTp wild type mostly exhibited astrocytic features, with a median OS of 57 months. Patients with both IDH1/IDH2 mutation and TERTp mutation typically demonstrated oligodendritic glial changes and had the best prognosis, with a median OS of 125 months.

The IDH1/IDH2 and TERTp mutations can aid in further classifying patients to guide treatment decisions. These markers not only help group patients based on their prognosis but also complement traditional histopathology to improve diagnostic accuracy. However, it is important to note that this study primarily focused on high-grade gliomas (HGG), and lower-grade gliomas were not extensively analyzed for prognosis and survival.

Our research findings suggest that combining TERTp and IDH mutation status can aid in further prognosis-related grouping of low-grade astrocytomas and 1p/19q intact lower-grade gliomas (LGGs). Similar to Hai Yan's study, the combination of TERTp and IDH mutations can aid in prognosis-related grouping of both high-grade gliomas (HGG) and LGG and potentially guide individualized treatment in the future.

Two significant clinical implications of molecular pathology are assessing prognosis and guiding treatment. The molecular pathological grouping of gliomas based on IDH/TERTp mutations is crucial in evaluating patients' prognosis, while IDH mutation plays a vital role in predicting the efficacy of adjuvant therapy. Given these findings, we further investigated whether combining TERTp mutations with IDH mutations could more accurately guide the comprehensive treatment of glioma. As a result, our research team at the Neurosurgery Department of Huashan Hospital, Fudan University, collaborated with Duke University and the Chinese University of Hong Kong to conduct a retrospective clinical study to explore this issue.

The study revealed that patients with IDHmut/TERTp mut, IDHmut/TERTpwt, and IDH wt/TERTpmut subtypes who received postoperative adjuvant therapy had significantly longer PFS than those without adjuvant therapy. Multifactorial survival analysis confirmed these results. However, in the IDH wt/TERTpwt subtype, no significant difference in PFS was observed between patients who received postoperative radiotherapy and those who did not. A typical case is presented in Fig. 9.1 to illustrate these findings.

The findings of this study suggest that TERTp mutation may provide complementary information to IDH mutation in predicting the sensitivity of patients with WHO grade II–III gliomas to postoperative adjuvant therapy. Specifically, further subclassifying IDH wild-type gliomas into IDHwt/TERTpmut and IDHwt/TERTpwt subtypes may help distinguish between patients who are likely to benefit from adjuvant therapy and those who are not. The former subtype showed sensitivity to adjuvant therapy, while the latter showed insensitivity. However, as this study is retrospective and has a relatively limited sample size, the conclusions should be confirmed by larger retrospective studies and clinical trials.

The CATNON trial, a phase III study utilizing a 2 × 2 analytic randomized design, enrolled 751 mesenchymal glioma patients without 1p/19q codeletion. These patients were treated with radiation therapy of 59.4 Gy, concurrent temozolomide (TMZ) with radiotherapy, 12 sequential cycles of TMZ after radiotherapy, or the Stupp regimen. Results presented at the 2019 American Society of Clinical Oncology meeting showed that the 5-year overall survival (OS) with or without concurrent TMZ was 50.2% (95% CI 44.4–55.7) and

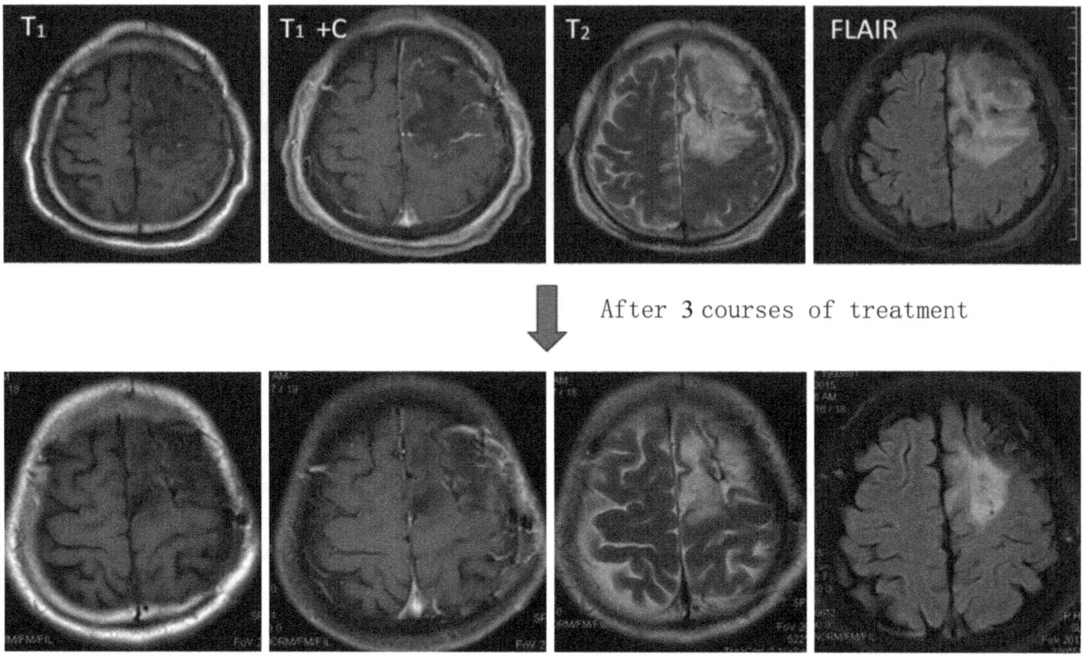

Fig. 9.1 Patient with recurrent astrocytoma (2016 version of WHO criteria) postoperatively, staged as IDH mut/TERTpwt, stable disease after 3 courses of cisplatin + TMZ adjuvant chemotherapy

52.7% (95% CI 46.9–58.1), respectively. The median OS of patients with IDH wild-type tumors was 19 months (95% CI 16.3–22.3), while the median OS of patients with IDH mutations was 116 months (95% CI 82.0–6.6). The IDH mutation status can predict the benefit of TMZ adjuvant chemotherapy, with a hazard ratio (HR) in the IDH mutation group of 0.41 (95% CI 0.27–0.64) and HR in the IDH wild-type group of 1.05 (95% CI 0.73–1.52); $p = 0.001$ for cross-test. In patients with IDH mutations treated with TMZ adjuvant therapy, the HR was 0.71 (95% CI 0.35–1.42, $p = 0.32$) for OS after concurrent TMZ treatment. The concurrent TMZ/radiotherapy group did not improve the OS in the study cohort, but there was a trend toward a survival benefit of concurrent TMZ/radiotherapy in patients with IDH-mutant tumors. Adjuvant TMZ treatment increased OS in patients with IDH-mutation tumors, while no additional OS benefit was observed in patients with IDH wild-type tumors.

In the RTOG9802 trial, researchers classified 106 patients (42%) into molecular subtypes, with 41% being IDHmut/non-co-deleted, 35% IDHmut/co-deleted, and 24% IDHwt. Results showed that patients with IDHmut/co-deleted and IDHmut/non-co-deleted subtypes had significantly prolonged PFS and OS after receiving PCV regimen, consistent with the results in RTOG9402 (JCO2014). However, patients with IDHwt subtype did not achieve significant survival benefits with PCV regimen.

In summary, there is a wealth of evidence from numerous clinical trials and retrospective studies based on molecular typing conducted in China and abroad. These studies provide valuable insights into the adjuvant treatment of glioma and are of great assistance to neurosurgeons, oncologists, and radiologists.

9.3 Molecular Targeted Therapy for Glioma

Angiogenesis, which is characterized by the growth of new blood vessels, is a critical feature of GBM and has been a focus of research in neuro-oncology for many years. Vascular endothelial growth factor (VEGF) and its receptor

VEGFR are the most important pro- and anti-angiogenic factors in this process. Bevacizumab, a human recombinant monoclonal antibody that binds to all VEGF isoforms, has been the first anti-angiogenic drug approved by the FDA for the treatment of recurrent GBM. Although previous studies have shown that bevacizumab can improve prognosis in colorectal, lung, breast, and kidney cancers, randomized clinical trials have not yet demonstrated prolonged overall survival (OS) for glioma patients. Studies have indicated that bevacizumab in combination with the oral alkylating agent lomustine may significantly prolong survival in patients with recurrent GBM compared to monotherapy. Phase II clinical trials have also shown that bevacizumab in combination with irinotecan can result in remission rates of up to 60% and a 6-month progression-free survival (PFS-6) of 38–46% in recurrent GBM patients. Another phase II trial compared bevacizumab in combination with irinotecan to bevacizumab alone for recurrent GBM, resulting in remission rates of 38% and 28% and PFS-6 of 50% and 42%, respectively. However, the efficacy of bevacizumab was not confirmed in a phase III trial for newly diagnosed GBM patients. The RTOG0825 trial was a controlled study that evaluated the use of bevacizumab (or placebo) in combination with standard concurrent radiotherapy and temozolomide (TMZ) regimens in patients with newly diagnosed GBM. The results indicated that the overall survival (OS) in the bevacizumab group was similar to that in the control group. Although the bevacizumab group had a longer progression-free survival (PFS) than the control group, the difference was not statistically significant.

With the growing importance of molecular markers in the management of glioma, it has become crucial to investigate whether different molecular markers can predict the efficacy of specific chemotherapies. For example, the status of MGMT promoter methylation can indicate sensitivity to TMZ chemotherapy. However, the prediction of chemotherapy efficacy by IDH/TERT mutations has been less studied. Most predictive studies based on IDH/TERT quadruplication are for conventional chemotherapy regimens (e.g., cisplatin + TMZ, or in combination with ACNU-based drugs), but not for anti-angiogenic drugs such as bevacizumab. Nonetheless, some glioma patients have shown efficacy with bevacizumab salvage therapy after failing conventional chemotherapy. The following case is a typical example.

This patient was diagnosed with giant cell GBM, with molecular typing revealing an IDH wild-type and TERT promoter wild-type status. After three cycles of cisplatin plus TMZ every 2 weeks, disease progression was confirmed by radiological images. However, partial remission was observed after a single course of bevacizumab and ACNU regimen (as shown in Fig. 9.2). Thus, we are currently investigating the potential prognostic value of IDH/TERT quadruplication on bevacizumab treatment for glioma, particularly for recurrent GBM. Furthermore, we aim to conduct a more comprehensive evaluation of the treatment effects using various multimodality imaging tools. Our clinical study suggests a potential trend toward better objective remission rates (ORR) in patients with recurrent HGG and MGMT promoter methylation and TERT promoter wild-type status who are treated with bevacizumab and nitrosoureas.

There are several drugs targeting VEGF that have been investigated in addition to bevacizumab. Cediranib, an oral VEGF inhibitor, showed some effect in a phase II single-center clinical trial but did not show a prolongation of PFS in phase III trials, either as a single agent or in combination with lomustine. Other drugs such as VEGF trap and enzastaurin have not shown significant effects. In contrast, EGFR-targeted drugs erlotinib and gefitinib showed little efficacy in recurrent GBM, and irreversible EGFR inhibitors like afatinib have also not shown sufficient efficacy. Currently, second-generation EGFR inhibitors such as dacomitinib and NCT01112527 are being investigated. Other targeted agents include the mammalian sirolimus-targeted inhibitor sirolimus and the farnesyltransferase inhibitor tipifarnib, which showed a modest effect in the treatment of recurrent GBM. Recent global clinical trials have emerged investigating inhibitors of

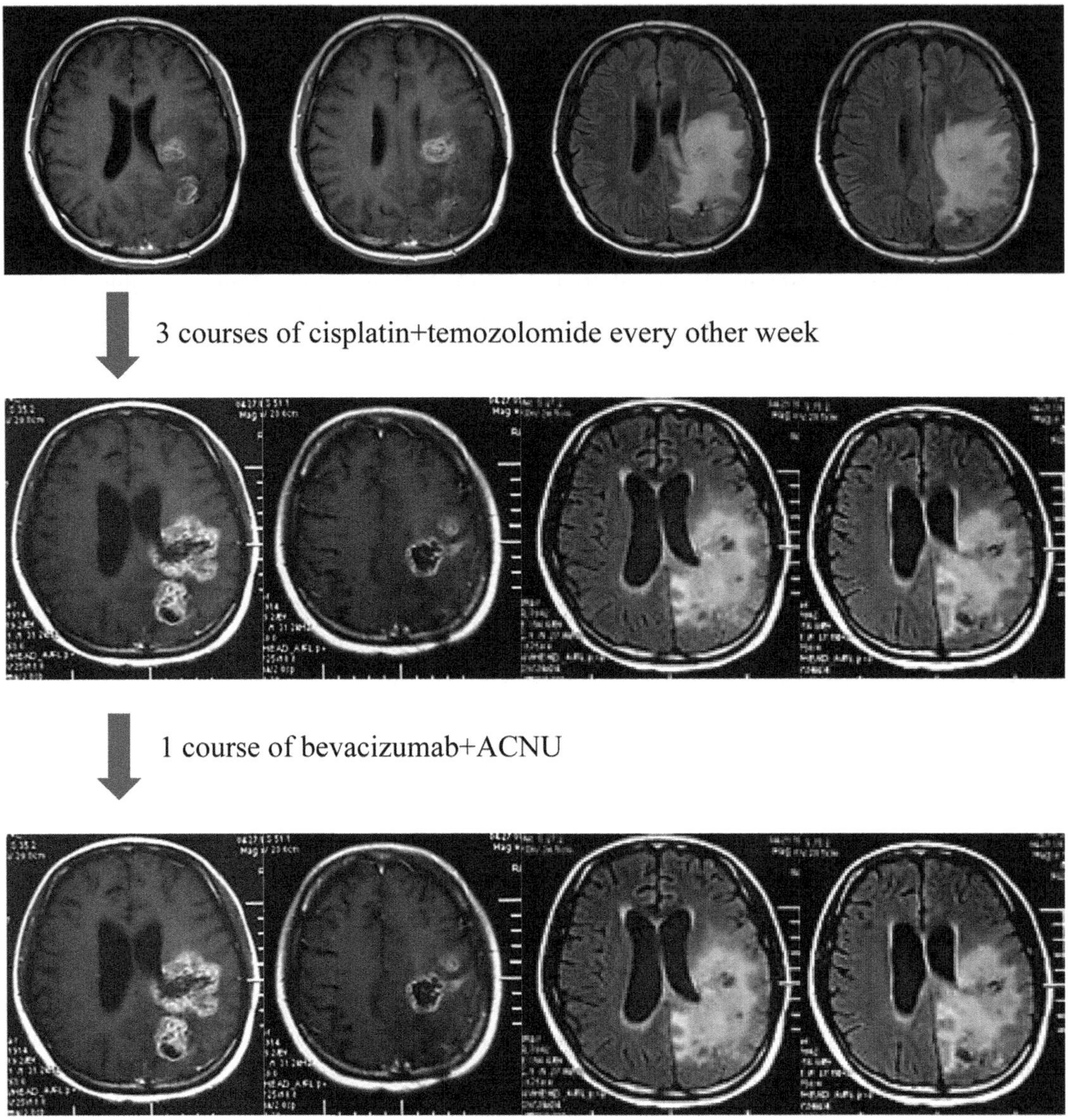

Fig. 9.2 One typical case of recurrent GBM treated with bevacizumab

mutant IDH, and some progress has been made. In a phase I clinical trial conducted in the United States, two inhibitors of mutant IDH, ivosidenib (AG-120) and vorasidenib (AG-881), were used for perioperative adjuvant treatment of patients with recurrent LGG with IDH mutations. The results showed that both AG-120 and AG-881 were effective in suppressing 2-HG levels in IDH1-mutated gliomas with more than 90% suppression compared to the control group, without significant adverse effects.

In summary, while diffuse glioma is still regarded as an incurable disease and GBM has a particularly dismal prognosis, recent progress in molecular pathology, high-throughput gene sequencing, and the selection of multiple chemotherapeutic/targeted agents are all paving the way for future success. It is our belief that combination therapy and individualized treatment regimens will be pivotal in the management of glioma.

Further Reading

Balana C, Barroso CM, Del Barco Berron S, et al. Randomized phase IIb clinical trial of continuation or non-continuation with six cycles of temozolomide after the first six cycles of standard first-line treatment in patients with glioblastoma: a Spanish research group in neuro-oncology (GEINO) trial. J Clin Oncol. 2019;37(15_suppl):2001.

Bell EH, Won M, Fleming JL, et al. Updated predictive analysis of the WHO-defined molecular subgroups of low-grade gliomas within the high-risk treatment arms of NRG Oncology/RTOG J 9802. Clin Oncol. 2019;37(15_suppl):2002.

Brennan CW, Verhaak RG, McKenna A, et al. The somatic genomic landscape of glioblastoma. Cell. 2013;155(2):462–77.

Cairncross G, Wang M, Shaw E, et al. Phase III trial of chemoradiotherapy for anaplastic oligodendroglioma: long-term results of RTOG J 9402. Clin Oncol. 2013;31(3):337–43.

Chan AK, Yao Y, Zhang Z, et al. TERT promoter mutations contribute to subset prognostication of lower-grade gliomas. Mod Pathol. 2015;28(2):177–86.

Dikang C, Ding Prim J, Zhang ZY, et al. Bevacizumab combined with nitrosoureas for the treatment of recurrent high: a Single-arm phase II clinical study of grade glioma. Chin J Cancer. 2018;28(9):649–56.

Gilbert MR, Dignam JJ, Armstrong TS, et al. A randomized trial of bevacizumab for newly diagnosed glioblastoma. N Engl J Med. 2014;370(8):699–708.

Hartmann C, Hentschel B, Wick W, et al. Patients with IDH1 wild type anaplastic astrocytomas exhibit worse prognosis than IDH1-mutated glioblastomas, and IDH1 mutation status accounts for the unfavorable prognostic effect of higher age: implications for classification of gliomas. Acta Neuropathol. 2010;120(6):707–18.

Houillier C, Wang X, Kaloshi G, et al. IDH1 or IDH2 mutations predict longer survival and response to temozolomide in low-grade gliomas. Neurology. 2010;75(17):1560–6.

Jones DT, Kocialkowski S, Liu L, et al. Tandem duplication producing a novel oncogenic BRAF fusion gene defines the majority of pilocytic astrocytomas. Cancer Res. 2008;68(21):8673–7.

Killela PJ, Reitman ZJ, Jiao Y, et al. TERT promoter mutations occur frequently in gliomas and a subset of tumors derived from cells with low rates of self renewal. Proc Natl Acad Sci USA. 2013;110(15):6021–6.

Killela PJ, Pirozzi CJ, Healy P, et al. Mutations in IDH1, IDH2, and in the TERT promoter define clinically distinct subgroups of adult malignant gliomas. Oncotarget. 2014;5(6):1515–25.

Louis DN, Perry A, Reifenberger G, et al. The 2016 World Health Organization classification of tumors of the central nervous system: a summary. Acta Neuropathol. 2016;131(6):803–20.

Mellinghoff IK, Cloughesy TF, Wen PY, et al. A phase I, open label, perioperative study of AG-120 and AG-881 in recurrent IDH1 mutant, low-grade glioma. Results from cohort 1. J Clin Oncol. 2019;37(15_suppl):2003.

Shaw EG, Wang M, Coons SW, et al. Randomized trial of radiation therapy plus procarbazine, lomustine, and vincristine chemotherapy for supratentorial adult low-grade glioma: initial results of RTOG 9802. J Clin Oncol. 2012;30(25):3065–70.

Songtao Q, Lei Y, Si G, et al. IDH mutations predict longer survival and response to temozolomide in secondary glioblastoma. Cancer Sci. 2012;103(2):269–73.

van den Bent MJ, Baumert B, Erridge SC, et al. Interim results from the CATNON trial (EORTC study 26053-22054) of treatment with concurrent and adjuvant temozolomide for 1p/19q non-co-deleted anaplastic glioma: a phase3, randomised, open-label intergroup study. Lancet. 2017;390(10103):1645–53.

Van Den Bent MJ, Erridge S, Vogelbaum MA, et al. Second interim and first molecular analysis of the EORTC randomized phase III intergroup CATNON trial on concurrent and adjuvant temozolomide in anaplastic glioma without 1p/19q codeletion. J Clin Oncol. 2019;37(15_suppl):2000.

Weller M, Le Rhun E, Preusser M, et al. How we treat glioblastoma. ESMO Open. 2019;4(Suppl 2):e000520.

Yan H, Parsons DW, Jin G, et al. IDH1 and IDH2 mutations in gliomas. N Engl J Med. 2009;360(8):765–73.

Zhang ZY, Chan AK, Ding XJ, et al. TERT promoter mutations contribute to IDH mutations in predicting differential responses to adjuvant therapies in WHO grade II and III diffuse gliomas. Oncotarget. 2015;6(28):24871–83.

10 Immunotherapy and Oncolytic Virus Would Provide New Adjuvant Therapy

Wei Hua

10.1 A Brief History of the Development of Tumor Immunotherapy

Tumor immunotherapy aims to stimulate and restore the body's natural immune response to recognize and attack tumor cells. This Goal can be achieved by activating or mobilizing the immune system or by infusing immune-active cells. In addition to traditional vaccines and antibodies, tumor immunotherapy now encompasses a range of approaches, including small molecule targeted drugs, cytokines, gene modifications, and other derivatives developed through various immunological methods. With the integration of modern biotechnology, tumor immunotherapy has emerged as the fourth mode of cancer treatment, alongside surgery, chemotherapy, and radiotherapy, known as tumor bioimmunotherapy. Malignant brain tumors are currently treated with surgery, radiotherapy, and chemotherapy, which can be described by patients as "sharp knives, branding irons, and poisons." Immunotherapy, in contrast, has fewer overall adverse effects, is more specific, and holds great potential for personalized treatment. As a result, immunotherapy has become a major area of research in translational medicine and an important practice for treating malignant brain tumors.

The development of modern tumor immunotherapy has been a long and challenging journey spanning over 100 years. In the late nineteenth century, orthopedic surgeon William Coley at the Sloan-Kettering Cancer Center observed tumor regression in osteosarcoma patients who had co-infections, which inspired him to experiment with injecting a bacterial mixture into osteosarcoma patients, marking the first modern attempt at tumor immunotherapy. However, the results were not satisfactory. In 1909, Paul Ehrlich proposed the theory of "immunosurveillance," which suggests that the immune system continuously patrols and destroys cancer cells. This theory was later systematized into the "immunosurveillance theory" by Thomas, Burnet, and Good. In the 1960s, monoclonal antibody technology was introduced, and M.S. Mahaley attempted to treat brain tumors with monoclonal antibodies. The 1970s saw a surge of nonspecific tumor immunotherapy, including bacillus Calmette-Guérin (BCG) and the serological determination of alpha-fetoprotein (AFP). Diagnostic and prognostic tumor markers such as AFP and carcinoembryonic antigen (CEA) also emerged. In 1973, R.M. Steinman discovered dendritic cells (DC), which became an essential vehicle for tumor immunotherapy. In the 1980s, advances in molecular biology, the development of transgenic mice, and recombinant cDNA expression library serum SEREX assays led to rapid progress in tumor immunity, with interleukin-2 (IL-2), interferon

W. Hua (✉)
Department of Neurosurgery, Huashan Hospital, Fudan University, Shanghai, China

Y. Mao (ed.), *Progress in the Diagnosis and Treatment of Gliomas*, Experts' Perspectives on Medical Advances, https://doi.org/10.1007/978-981-99-0123-4_10

(IFN), and sequential immunotherapy being applied to various malignancies. However, most of these attempts failed in phase II/III clinical trials, and the relationship between tumor and immunity was highly controversial. Nevertheless, these failures led to a better understanding of the human immune system. In the early 1990s, breakthroughs were made in the study of antigen presentation and T-cell recognition mechanisms, and recombinant genetic technologies and humanized genetically engineered antibodies were gradually introduced into clinical applications. As of 2008, the FDA has approved over 20 tumor immunotherapy products, including monoclonal antibodies (e.g., anti-VEGF monoclonal antibody bevacizumab), immune adjuvants (e.g., BCG, TLR agonist imiquimod, etc.), cytokines (e.g., IFN-α, IL-2, TNF-α, etc.), adjuvant drugs (e.g., GM-CSF, etc.), and prophylactic vaccines (e.g., HBV, HPV vaccines, etc.). In April 2010 and March 2011, the FDA approved Sipuleucel-T and ipilimumab, respectively, for advanced estrogen therapy-naïve prostate cancer and advanced melanoma. Ipilimumab is a CTLA-4 antagonist that inhibits the negative regulation of T cells, making it easier for cytotoxic T lymphocytes (CTLs) to destroy melanoma cells. These immunotherapeutic products have shown to be effective, although there are some problems with them. Their successful launch marks a new stage in the clinical application of tumor immunotherapy. In recent years, the development of tumor immunotherapy has been rapidly changing, and tumor immunity has entered a new era. Immunological theories and methods have been widely used in tumor diagnosis and treatment, and the scope of tumor immunotherapy is still expanding. Immunological methods are evolving as a tool to combat cancer.

Immunotherapy was once considered the sword of Damocles in the battle against cancer, but with its development, researchers have encountered challenges in fully understanding the complexity of human immunity. On the other hand, this has led to the resurgence of immunology, unraveling many mysteries and opening up a new era of tumor immunotherapy. While certain malignancies, like melanoma and prostate cancer, have shown promising results in immunotherapy, there are still many cancers, including gliomas, that require further investigation in this field. The CNS is known to lack a typical lymphatic drainage system. Normally, T cells are virtually absent from the CNS, but they can enter in large numbers in response to inflammation. Despite the theory being widely accepted, little is known about how immune cells enter and exit the CNS. Due to its highly immune-tolerant nature, brain tumor immunity is unique. However, with the development of CNS immunity, the CNS has been recognized as an "immune-specific" rather than an "immune-privileged" organ. This shift in understanding has been prompted by the discovery of CNS lymphatic vessels, which has changed the previous view. Antoine Louveau and colleagues made a groundbreaking discovery of functional lymphatic structures in the dural sinus when investigating the pathways of T cells in and out of the meninges. These lymphatic duct structures express all the molecular signatures of normal lymphatic duct endothelium and have the crucial function of transporting cerebrospinal fluid and lymphocytes. Furthermore, the lymphatic structures are also connected to deep cervical lymph nodes. This discovery has revolutionized the field of neuroimmunology and immunotherapy, paving the way for novel therapeutic approaches in treating neurodegenerative and inflammatory diseases. T-cell infiltration is also a common occurrence in gliomas, and the blood-brain barrier around malignant gliomas is often permeable to immune cells due to factors such as upregulated expression of aquaporins 4. Microglia in the central nervous system exhibits dendritic cell-like functions, which highlights the importance of CNS immunity in brain tumors, inflammatory and autoimmune diseases, degenerative diseases, and the development of gliomas. In the early stages of malignant brain tumors, host immunity is minimally affected, making immunotherapy an attractive option. Serum levels of IFN-γ, IL-17, IL-6, IL-23, TGF-β, among others, in patients with different grades of glioma, are not significantly different from those of normal controls. However, malignant glioma has been shown to suppress host immunity by reducing the number of CD3, CD4, and NK cells, causing an imbalance in the CD4/CD8 ratio, and decreasing IgG, IgM, and IgA in the host serum. To effectively prevent and treat malignant brain tumors, we need a better understanding of CNS immunity and identify suitable strategies to engage the body's immune system.

Tumor immunotherapy can be classified into different types based on the methods used, such as nonspecific and specific immunity, passive immunity, and active immunity. Nonspecific immunity includes cytokines, BCG therapy, etc. Specific immunotherapy includes specific antigenic peptides, antibodies, and T-cell immunotherapy loaded with specific antigens. Passive immunity involves the importation of exogenous immune response factors to enhance the body's anti-tumor immune response for the purpose of tumor treatment, such as monoclonal antibody targeted therapy and relay transfusion of lymphocytes. Active immunity uses tumor antigens to stimulate the body to generate specific immune responses to prevent tumor growth, spread, and recurrence, such as antigenic peptide vaccines, genetically modified vaccines, and anti-unique antibodies. These methods include monoclonal antibody therapy, vaccines, secondary immunotherapy, and cytokine therapy. However, according to current research, single-agent immunotherapy is not very effective, and combination therapy strategies are often used, such as combining DC and relay T cells, using antigenic adjuvants, synchronizing immunotherapy and suppression of immune escape, and combining immunotherapy with radiotherapy. In the following sections, we will analyze brain tumor immunotherapy from different perspectives.

10.2 Glioma Tumor-Associated Antigens Are a Difficult and Important Focus of Current Research

Tumor antigens play a crucial role in activating the body's anti-tumor immune response and are therefore key to successful immunotherapy. The discovery of the mechanism of tumor antigen recognition in the 1990s paved the way for specific active immunotherapy. Through this approach, the genes encoding more than 10 tumor-specific antigens, including MAGE-3, MART-1, and Tyrosinase, have been successfully cloned. In 2005, the National Cancer Institute launched The Cancer Genome Atlas (TCGA) project, which aimed to provide a deeper understanding of tumors. GBM was the first tumor type to be selected and its results have greatly advanced our knowledge of brain tumor immunology.

Tumor antigens can be classified into two categories: tumor-specific antigens (TSAs) and tumor-associated antigens (TAAs). Although malignant tumors share some common properties, only a few of their proteins have been found to be common to all tumors. Tumor proteomics has identified 8 common proteins, including RhoGDI, vimentin, ATP synthase, cathepsin D precursor, enolase1, peroxiredoxin1, annexin4, and HSP27. While these proteins play some role in the immune response, they are not particularly immunogenic. Many glioma-associated antigens have been reported in the literature, such as IL-13 receptor alpha2 chain, EphA2, gp100, gp240, tenascin, T lymphocyte-recognized squamous cell carcinoma antigen Sart, and WDR. However, the heterogeneity of gliomas makes these antigens poor representatives. In the following section, we will provide examples of some antigens associated with brain tumors.

EGFRv III: EGFR gene amplification and overexpression are found in 40% of primary GBM cases, particularly in the "classic" molecular subtypes. About half of these cases are accompanied by EGFR mutations, with type III EGFR mutations being the most common. The EGFRvIII mutation can activate MAPK and PI3K signaling pathways, leading to tumor cell proliferation, angiogenesis, and resistance to radiotherapy. A peptide vaccine called CDX-110 has been developed to target EGFRvIII, and a phase II clinical trial showed that a peptide antigen conjugated with an adjuvant called keyhole limpet hemocyanin (KLH) improved the progression-free survival (PFS) of GBM patients. However, EGFRvIII disappeared after most tumor recurrence, suggesting the need for further exploration of immune escape mechanisms. Cancer-testis antigen (CTA) is a group of tumor-associated antigens with specific expression patterns that share common features. These include (1) expression in normal tissues that is restricted to germ cells of testes, ova, and trophoblast cells of the placenta, while expression in various tumor tissues occurs at different frequencies; (2) most CT antigens are located on the X chromosome, including MAGE, GAGE, and NY-ESO-1, with only a few located on other chromosomes such as SCP-1; (3) they are usually found in multiple family members; and (4) CT antigen expression is often heterogeneous in tumor tissues of various origins. Therefore, CTA is well characterized as a tumor-associated antigen. MAGE-1 is expressed in gliomas and has been used as a marker to evaluate the anti-glioma immune response. Additionally, MAGE-2 is highly expressed in medulloblastoma and ventricular meningioma, while SSX-4 is expressed in oligodendroglioma. The IDH mutation is not expressed in normal brain tissue but only in tumors and is therefore considered a promising target for immunotherapy. Currently, clinical trials for IDH mutation inhibitors and vaccines against IDH mutations are underway.

Despite the advancements in technology, the search for glioma antigens remains a challenge. In a review of 58 glioma proteomics studies, Kalinina et al. found inconsistent results across different research groups, indicating the absence of a common gene or protein as a glioma-specific biomarker. Tumor heterogeneity further complicates this issue. The lack of tumor-specific antigens is a major obstacle in immunotherapy for malignant tumors, where tumor antigens play a crucial role in antitumor immunity. However, identifying tumor antigens not only helps to unravel the molecular mechanisms of tumor immunity but also establishes the basis for developing new methods of tumor immunological diagnosis and prevention.

After malignant transformation, tumor cells produce antigenic proteins that are degraded intracellularly. Certain short peptides resulting from the degradation process can bind to MHC class I molecules in the endoplasmic reticulum and be presented on the cell surface, a process known as antigen processing and presentation. T cells play a crucial role in anti-tumor immunity, and their activation and effector stages are well studied. The first signal for T-cell activation is provided by the binding of an antigen-specific receptor (TCR) on the surface of T cells and an MHC-antigen peptide complex on the surface of APC or tumor cells. The second signal is generated by the binding of costimulatory molecules (such as CD80/CD86) on APC cells and the corresponding receptors (such as CD28) on the surface of T cells. Another pathway involves B7H2 binding to ICOS to generate positive costimulatory signals, while B7-H1 binding to PD-1 stimulates negative costimulatory signals. CTLA-4 and B7H1 are sites in the antigen presentation process that can be targeted to achieve anti-tumor immune effects.

10.3 General Immunotherapies for Glioma

Tumor vaccines aim to stimulate the body's immune response against tumors as a way to treat them. The application of modern molecular technology in the early 1980s gave rise to a new generation of vaccines, revitalizing the development of tumor vaccines. Antibody technology has also progressed from the initial immunization of animals to the third generation of genetically engineered antibodies, and various cytokines have been identified. Although successive immunotherapies have taken time to develop, researchers have combined different approaches over the years, resulting in numerous anti-tumor immunotherapy options. This section highlights several important anti-brain tumor immunotherapies, including monoclonal antibody-targeted therapies, peptide vaccines, DC vaccines, secondary immunotherapy, and cytokine therapy. These bio-immunotherapies have demonstrated efficacy in removing small metastases and occult foci following surgery, preventing tumor metastasis and recurrence, and causing fewer adverse effects overall. As a result, they are ideal adjuvant therapies after surgery.

(1) Monoclonal antibody-targeted therapy: In 1975, Kohler and Milstein developed a B-cell hybridoma cell line by fusing immunized mouse spleen cells with myeloma cells, resulting in the production of monoclonal antibodies. The hybridoma technique propelled the development of anti-tumor antibodies, but these antibodies also had limitations. They were more suited for diagnostic purposes and less effective for therapeutic use. With the advent of genetically engineered antibodies, in vitro high-capacity cell culture, computer-controlled production, and the Human Genome Project breakthrough, a range of modern biotechnologies emerged, including genomics, proteomics, bioinformatics, and biochip technologies. This led to the continuous improvement of monoclonal antibodies, which are the most commonly used targeting molecules. The new generation of small molecule targeted drugs are more specific and have a lower molecular weight, making them more likely to enter the target area and bind to tumor cells. However, their effects may not be exclusively immunological. Furthermore, molecularly targeted drug research has been expedited by computerized virtual screening, combinatorial chemistry, and high-throughput screening.

In the 1960s, Mahaley attempted to treat brain tumors using monoclonal antibodies, but more recent studies have combined monoclonal antibodies with factors such as isotopes and chemotherapeutic agents in an attempt to target tumors. However, the results have been unsatisfactory. Monoclonal antibodies can target both tumor-specific antigen (TAA) and non-TAA, and their anti-tumor effects can be classified into direct and indirect effects. Direct effects include antibody-dependent cell-mediated cytotoxicity (ADCC), complement-dependent cytotoxicity (CDC), and McAb active immunity. The direct action on TAA is the most important. Indirect effects occur when monoclonal antibodies bind to isotopes, chemotherapeutic agents, or toxins to reach the tumor and exert anti-tumor effects. Small-molecule targeted drugs are mostly classified as chemotherapeutic drugs, but they are also closely related to immunity. They are monoclonal antibody molecules that target signaling pathways and can be classified into receptor tyrosine kinases and non-receptor tyrosine kinases, as well as single-target inhibitors and multi-target inhibitors. Here, we present several classical targeted drugs against malignant brain tumors as examples.

CTLA-4 antibody (ipilimumab): The CTLA-4 antibody (ipilimumab) was approved by the FDA in 2011 for the treatment of melanoma. CTLA-4 negatively regulates anti-tumor immunity, and this antibody blocks the negative regulation, allowing T cells to destroy tumor cells more easily. PD1 is structurally similar to CTLA-4 but has different functions. CTLA-4 activates primary T cells, whereas PD1 inhibits activated T cells. Additionally, the PD1 ligands, PDL1 and PDL2, are mainly expressed in the tumor microenvironment. Tumor cells induce inhibitory receptors PDL1 and PDL2 in response to immune attack, a mechanism known as adaptive drug resistance. The anti-PD1 monoclonal antibody could theoretically address this challenge. However, these two new classes of immunotherapy products have not yet been used in glioma treatment. Many other antibodies have shown promising results in animal studies, but further clinical trials are necessary to verify their effectiveness in humans.

Anti-EGFR monoclonal antibodies: Monoclonal antibodies targeting EGFR have been the focus of research as EGFR plays a critical role in the growth of tumors, including malignant gliomas. Trastuzumab (Herceptin) is used for HER2 receptor-overexpressed breast cancer, cetuximab (Erbitux) for HER-1-positive metastatic colorectal cancer, and gefitinib (Iressa) and erlotinib (Tarceva) for advanced non-small cell lung cancer (NSCLC) with HER-2 receptor overexpression. Although small-molecule EGFR tyrosine kinase inhibitors are effective in breast, colorectal, and lung cancers, they are not effective in improving PFS in patients with malignant gliomas. Lapatinib and cetuximab, the HER2 inhibitor and anti-EGFR monoclonal antibody, respectively, are also ineffective against malignant brain tumors. Nitrozumab (nimotuzumab) is another humanized anti-EGFR monoclonal antibody currently in clinical trials for the treatment of brain tumors.

Anti-angiogenesis drugs: Anti-angiogenic drugs have been developed to target tumor angiogenesis, which is closely related to VEGF. VEGF binds to the receptor VEGFR, activating the classical MAPK and PI3K signaling pathways and promoting angiogenesis. Other signaling pathways, including angiopoietin, hypoxia-inducible factor (HIF), and DLL4/Notch, are also involved in tumor angiogenesis. Avastin was approved by the US FDA in 2008 for the treatment of breast cancer and has shown efficacy in the treatment of rectal cancer, ocular neovascularization and exudative lesions, and necrosis and edema after radiation therapy for malignant gliomas. However, the FDA re-evaluated Avastin in 2010 and withdrew its approval for breast cancer due to a lack of survival benefit. In a phase I clinical trial in malignant glioma, Avastin prolonged progression-free survival (PFS), and the combination of Avastin and Irinotecan, a new generation of phase S cell cycle-specific chemotherapy, significantly improved PFS and overall survival (OS) in patients with malignant glioma. However, further clinical trials are needed to confirm these results. Additionally, the pro-tumorigenic effect of hepatocyte growth factor (HGF) depends on the phosphorylation of MET. Therefore, anti-VEGF treatment weakens the inhibition of the HGF signaling pathway by VEGF and may enhance the proliferation and metastasis of glioma cells. The combination of bevacizumab and sorafenib has been used, but the improvement of OS in malignant glioma is not significant. Anti-angiogenic targeted drugs may need to be combined with chemotherapy or other signaling pathway inhibitors to achieve optimal outcomes.

STAT-3: STAT-3 is a transcription factor that plays a crucial role in tumor proliferation, anti-apoptosis, angiogenesis, and immune escape. In normal physiological conditions, STAT-3 activation is triggered by ligand-receptor interactions, mainly through growth factor receptor tyrosine kinase, cytokine, and G-protein receptor pathways. In malignant brain tumors, EGFR, EGFRvIII, and IL-6 activate Jak2, which then phosphorylates STAT-3 to activate it. Additionally, STAT-3 has immunosuppressive effects by preventing DC maturation and inhibiting macrophage activation. Inhibitors of STAT-3 have also been found to upregulate CD80 and CD86 co-stimulatory molecules of microglia in the central nervous system, inducing activation and proliferation of T cells. WP1066 is a small molecule inhibitor of STAT-3 that has multiple immunomodulatory functions and is considered an emerging drug for future immunotherapy.

Other: The PI3K/AKT/mTOR signaling pathway is a downstream target of EGFR, and although small molecule inhibitors targeting mTOR, such as sirolimus and its derivatives, have been investigated for the treatment of malignant brain tumors, they appear to be less effective. The efficacy of farnesyltransferase inhibitors, such as tipifarnib and lonafarnib, also needs further investigation. Thalidomide, an inhibitor of bFGF and VEGF signaling pathways, has shown modest anti-malignant glioma effects. Cyclooxygenase-2 inhibitors and matrix metalloproteinase (MMP) inhibitors targeting tumor invasion are currently undergoing clinical trials to evaluate their anti-brain tumor effects. Due to the complexity of the signaling pathway, it is difficult to target a single pathway to inhibit tumors, and combination therapy with multiple pathway-targeted drugs may become the future direction for the treatment of malignant brain tumors.

(2) Peptide vaccines: The aggressive growth of gliomas has made the development of novel therapies urgent, as many current treatments are unavailable. However, we know that the immune system can be used to fight tumors, despite the blood-brain barrier separating the central nervous system. Antigenic peptides can directly stimulate the body's immune system or be used to prepare various vaccines, such as peptide/protein vaccines, nucleic acid (DNA) vaccines, tumor cell vaccines, DC vaccines, genetic vaccines, engineered recombinant vaccines, hybrid vaccines, MHC antigen-peptide combination vaccines, HSP-peptide combination vaccines, and peptide vaccine and adjuvant combinations. The EGFRv III peptide vaccine is a relatively successful case, which has entered the phase III clinical stage, and the efficacy is being further observed. Moreover, some authors have combined multiple TAA antigenic peptides to preserve immunogenicity and compensate for the weak expression of individual antigens. Okada prepared a DC vaccine for recurrent glioma by combining EphA2, IL-13Rα2, YKL-40, and gp100 414 antigens. These antigenic peptides can be mixed to produce a vaccine for personalized treatment.

Tumor vaccines can target either tumor-specific peptide antigens or tumor-associated antigens. Recent studies have focused on developing vaccines targeting tumor-specific antigens, such as EGFRv III and IDH1 mutations. EGFRv III mutant proteins are a result of tumor-specific splicing of EGFR protein gene exons and account for approximately 20% of GBM cases. Although EGFRv III-targeted vaccines are currently in phase III clinical trials for first and recurrent GBM, their use is limited to a small proportion of glioma patients. While the IDH1 vaccine targets IDH1 protein mutations in LGG and recurrent GBM. A pilot study conducted by a group from the University of Heidelberg tested the IDH-vac vaccine on 32 patients with IDH1 mutated gliomas. The study found that the vaccine was effective in 27 patients (84.4%), and the PFS and OS of 3 years were 0.63 (95% CI 0.44 0.77) and 0.84 (95% CI 0.67 0.93), respectively. However, it is noteworthy that 12 patients (37.5%) in this cohort showed pseudo-progression, which was accompanied by higher T cells in the peripheral blood. To accurately assess these results, new neuroradiologic indices like iRANO may need to be introduced.

(3) DC vaccines: Dendritic cells (DCs) are a highly effective type of antigen-presenting cell and are commonly used in immunotherapy. DCs are derived from mononuclear cells in peripheral blood or bone marrow and are induced into DCs by GM-CSF and IL-4. A systematic review of current clinical trials investigating oncology DC vaccines shows that DC vaccines are safe and feasible for the treatment of glioma, with most trials observing prolonged progression-free survival (PFS) or overall survival (OS) in patients. For instance, Yu et al. reported a phase I clinical trial of acid-eluting antigen for the treatment of malignant glioma, where the mean survival of the immunotherapy group was 133 weeks, compared to only 30 weeks for the control group. Patients who underwent reoperation had memory T-cell and CD8+ T-cell infiltration in their tumors. The longest follow-up time was reported by Chang Gung Memorial Hospital, where 17 patients with recurrent and newly diagnosed malignant glioma were treated with a DC vaccine. The median OS of this group was 520 days, longer than the control group's 380 days, and the 5-year survival rate increased from 0 to 18.8% in the control group.

As specific antigens are lacking in glioma, mixed antigens are currently used more often in clinical practice. Along with tumor cell lysates, DC seedlings can be prepared by fusing tumor cells with DCs or by using total RNA from tumor cells. Studies have found that apoptotic cell-loaded DCs stimulate the best immune response from killer T cells and nonspecific NK cells. In our neurosurgery department, we have been experimenting with mixed antigens from glioma tumor stem cells (TSCs), referred to as "stem cell-like antigens," which have been shown to be more immunogenic than traditional mixed antigens. The stem cell-like antigens were prepared using a serum-free stem cell culture method to produce glioma stem cell spheres, and the killing rate of glioma cells by the stem cell-like antigen-mediated effector T cells was found to be significantly better than the traditional method in in vitro experiments. Both animal experiments and phase I clinical trials have confirmed the effectiveness of stem cell-like antigen-based anti-glioma immunotherapy. Further extraction and preparation of stem cell-like antigens using X-ray irradiation and CD133 sorting are more effective. In 2022, Linda M. Liau reported the results of a phase 3 prospective non-randomized clinical trial of autologous tumor lysate-loaded DC vaccination in GBM. The trial found that DCVax-L could significantly prolong OS in both newly diagnosed and recurrent GBM patients. Specifically, the OS was extended to 19.3 months in newly diagnosed GBM and 13.2 months in recurrent GBM, which were significantly better than their respective control groups. With the development of tumor stem cell theory and research, stem cell-like antigens hold promise for breaking the deadlock for immunotherapy of glioma.

Despite the relatively high safety profile of DC vaccines, their clinical responses in oncology remain limited due to factors such as the maturation status of DCs, the extent of subsequent lymphocyte induction, and the small number of exogenously loaded antigenic epitopes. To address these limitations, genetic modifications can be made to enhance the expression of tumor antigens and immunostimulatory molecules, cytokines, or chemokines that boost the immune response, as well as to downregulate immune-negative regulatory molecules. Numerous clinical trials have used subcutaneous or intramuscular injections of DC vaccines, and there is no significant evidence to suggest that different injection sites significantly affect their efficacy. However, there is a higher risk of adverse effects, such as cerebral edema, with tumor cavity injection. Prins et al. examined the gene expression of DC vaccine-treated gliomas and found that mesenchymal GBM exhibited greater sensitivity to immunotherapy and prolonged patient survival.

(4) Adoptive immunotherapy: Adoptive immunotherapy is a promising approach to treating tumors, utilizing autologous or donor lymphocytes that are immune to tumors. These cells are activated and expanded in vitro before being transfused into patients to enhance their anti-tumor immune response and prevent recurrence. The application of adoptive immunotherapy to anti-tumor research was inspired by the discovery of cellular immunity's involvement in tissue organ transplantation rejection in the 1960s. Lymphokine-activated killer cells (LAKs), discovered by Rosenberg in 1985, were found to have anti-tumor effects when expanded in vitro with high doses of IL-2. In 1986, Rosenberg also reported using IL-2 to expand tumor-infiltrating lymphocytes (TILs) for tumor treatment. In 1991, Schmidt at Stanford University discovered cytokine-induced killer cells (CIKs). In 2002, NCI researchers found that CD4+ T cells were essential in triggering an effective anti-tumor immune response, giving the order to attack to CD8+ T cells, the "soldiers" on the killing mission. In 2008, researchers at the MD Anderson Center successfully treated a patient with advanced melanoma using intravenously amplified CD4+ T cells loaded with the NY-ESO-1 antigen. In 2010, Sipuleucel-T was approved by the FDA for the treatment of advanced prostate cancer, which uses DC combined with T-cell immunotherapy.

LAK cells: Lymphokine-activated killer (LAK) cells have a broad-spectrum, MHC has non-restricted anti-tumor activity, and their main effector cells are CD56 and CD16. The efficacy of LAK cells against tumors is also influenced by their distribution in the tissues and organs after transfusion, with notable responses observed against melanoma, renal cell carcinoma, malignant lymphoma, ovarian cancer, and colon cancer. Since the 1980s, many researchers have attempted to use LAK cells to treat brain tumors, but the results have been limited, and adverse effects such as cerebral edema are common.

TIL cells: Tumor-infiltrating lymphocytes (TILs) are obtained by isolating cells from surgically resected tumor tissue, and then activating them in vitro through IL-2 induction. These cells are screened for IFN-γ-positive clones, which are then expanded to obtain lymphocytes with anti-tumor activity. TILs have MHC-restricted, tumor-specific killer cells and express CD3+CD8+ or CD3+CD4+ markers. In vitro studies have shown that TILs have a 100-fold greater anti-tumor effect than LAK cells with the same number of cells, but in vivo studies have not shown a significant increase in their anti-tumor effect. The presence of a wide variety of lymphocytes, including negative immunomodulatory cells such as Tregs, makes the screening of positive clones challenging.

CD3AK cells (anti-CD3McAbactivatedkillercells): CD3AK cells are a type of immune cell that contain a high proportion of CD3+CD56+ lymphocytes. These cells are capable of selectively killing tumor cells and have superior proliferative capacity compared to LAK cells. Additionally, CD3AK cells are less reliant on IL-2 and have been investigated for their potential use in brain tumor research.

CIK: CIK cells are generated through the co-culture of mononuclear cells from either peripheral blood or bone marrow with a range of cytokines including IL-2, IFN-γ, PHA, and anti-CD3 monoclonal antibodies. This process induces activation and efficient expansion of the cells, and phase I clinical trials are currently underway. Some researchers have also produced DC-CIK cells by co-culturing CIK cells with homologous DC cells. This approach promotes the maturation of DC cells and the proliferation of CIK cells, resulting in enhanced anti-tumor activity.

EALL cells (expanding activated autologous lymphocytes): It is a novel treatment approach that involves the expansion of killer lymphocytes, which primarily consist of CD8+ T cells and NK cells. CD8+ T cells, also known as CTL, target and eliminate tumor cells, while NK cells target tumor cells with downregulated HLA expression. The effectiveness of EALL treatment can vary based on factors such as the number of infusions, the type of disease being treated, and individual patient differences.

LAK cells and IL-2: Initial studies have shown that intra-tumoral injection of LAK cells and IL-2 can be effective in treating gliomas, although LAK cells are not highly specific to this type of tumor. Regardless of the method used to prepare effector cells, there are several challenges that arise after cell infusion, including adverse effects from pretreatment and adjuvant drugs, short retention time of effector cells in vivo, transient immune response, and the immunosuppressive effects of the tumor microenvironment. These factors can limit the clinical efficacy of this therapy and hinder the promotion of relay immunotherapy. However, combination therapies and new technologies hold promise for advancing secondary immunotherapy, which has emerged as a fast-developing approach in recent years.

CAR-T therapy: CAR-T therapy is a promising and increasingly popular approach to T-cell immunotherapy. This method involves genetic engineering to recombine antibody fragments of tumor-associated antigens with T-cell activation motifs, which are then introduced into T lymphocytes in peripheral blood using a virus as a carrier. The resulting tumor-specific T cells are called chimeric antigen receptor T cells (CAR-T). Second- and third-generation CAR-T therapies have been developed, which not only chimerize antigens but also incorporate co-stimulatory molecules to enhance the immune response. While CAR-T therapy has shown efficacy in treating other malignancies, its use in the treatment of gliomas is still in its early stages but holds great promise. However, as the number of clinical trials for CAR-T therapy increases, concerns about safety are also growing. These include the risk of insertional mutations, cytokine release syndrome, and off-target effects. As a result, maximizing the benefits of CAR-T therapy while minimizing potential risks and avoiding cytokine storms is a critical consideration that must be addressed.

The common targets for CAR-T therapy include IL13Rα2, EGFRvIII, HER2, and GD2. MUC1, CD147, and MMP2 are also potential targets. In 2016, an intrathecal injection of CAR-T therapy targeting IL13Rα2 successfully salvaged a relapsed, multifocal GBM patient. In 2022, GD2-CAR-T therapy demonstrated surprising clinical benefits in H3K27M DIPG and DMG patients, with 9 out of 10 patients showing radiological and/or clinical relief.

(5) Cytokine therapy: Cytokines play a crucial role in regulating the immune system, and the FDA has approved several cytokines such as IL-2, IFN-α, TNF-α, and GM-CSF for clinical use. Here is a brief overview of some commonly used anti-tumor cytokines.

IL-2: In 1976, IL-2 was identified by Morgan as a factor that promotes and maintains T-cell growth in vitro in mouse spleen cell culture supernatant. The combination of IL-2 and LAK cells has achieved certain efficacy in the treatment of advanced tumor patients, which has stimulated a great interest in the biological function of IL-2 and its clinical application. IL-2 does not directly kill tumor cells but rather stimulates and activates its effector cells to exert indirect antitumor effects. Melanoma and renal cell carcinoma are the most sensitive tumors treated with IL-2, while other tumors that respond to IL-2 treatment include breast cancer, ovarian cancer, colon cancer, small cell lung cancer, lymphoma, and acute myeloid leukemia. However, the remission period is usually not durable. In the case of glioma tumors, IL-2 is used in combination with NK cells, LAK cells, and TIL cells and is usually injected directly into the tumor cavity with a return infusion of activated lymphocytes. In some animal studies, the introduction of IL-4 and IL-2 into the tumor significantly suppressed tumor growth and prolonged the survival of tumor-bearing rats. The main adverse effects of IL-2 are fever and neurotoxicity, such as drowsiness, impaired consciousness, and cerebral edema.

IFN: IFN is a natural defense substance in the body that can be classified into α, β, and γ types, with a wide range of biological effects. IFN-α and IFN-β have potent antiviral effects, while IFN-γ is the main factor regulating the immune system. The antitumor ability of IFN arises from two aspects: (1) direct inhibition of tumor cell growth by inhibiting DNA synthesis and prolonging the cell cycle and (2) enhancement of the cytotoxicity of T cells and the killing power of NK cells and macrophages, thereby inhibiting tumor cells. IFN also has immune-modifying and immune-stimulatory effects, promoting the expression of MAGE-1 in malignant glioma, disclosing MHC antigenic epitopes, and upregulating MHC expression. Clinical trials have shown the efficacy of IFN-α in treating hairy cell leukemia and chronic myeloid leukemia and IFN-γ in treating non-Hodgkin's lymphoma, melanoma, and renal cell carcinoma. IFNs have been shown to inhibit the growth of gliomas, with IFN-α more commonly used as adjuvant therapy given systemically or locally, while the efficacy of IFN-β is still debated. IFN-β has been used clinically in malignant gliomas and recurrent gliomas with some success, but this response is of shorter duration. IFN-γ also has anti-tumor effects but has mostly been used in combination with other therapies. In animal studies by Yu et al., the co-introduction of IFN-γ and TNF-α into tumors using adenoviral vectors significantly inhibited tumor growth.

TNF-α and TNF-γ: TNF-α has demonstrated a significant anti-glioma effect and is effective in treating recurrent gliomas, whereas TNF-γ is less effective and less commonly used for glioma treatment. The use of cytokines alone in glioma therapy has become less frequent due to their high adverse effects, short half-life, low concentration in the tumor area, and poor efficacy. Nowadays, they are mostly used as targets for gene therapy or genetic engineering. Numerous studies have been conducted to introduce cytokine genes into the body via different vectors, allowing for a slow release of small amounts of cytokines locally in tumors to enhance efficacy and reduce systemic adverse effects. For example, in one study, P53, IL-2, IL-12, and cowpox virus were used as vectors for treating mice with glioma, resulting in a significant increase in peripheral blood NK cells, Mac-1+ cells, NKT cells, and tumor cells expressing IFN-γ and TNF-α, which inhibited the growth of tumor cells. Other cytokines, such as IL-6, IL-4, IL-12, IL-1β, and GM-CSF, have also been used in tumor immunotherapy. However, given the diversity of biological roles that cytokines play and their involvement in a complex network, understanding their relationship with disease onset and development is a challenging task. As a result, more research is needed to fully comprehend the therapeutic potential of cytokines in vivo and determine how to utilize them optimally.

(6) Other: Immune adjuvants, such as CpG oligodeoxynucleotides (TLR-9 agonist) and imiquimod (TLR-7 agonist), can enhance the immune response. In addition, CMV-associated antigen-mediated DC vaccines have been used in conjunction with the tetanus vaccine to increase CCL3 chemokines, assist DC cell homing, and enhance antitumor immunity. In a study published in Nature in March 2015, this approach showed some efficacy in clinical patients.

10.4 Immune Escape of Glioma Dramatically Impacts Immunotherapy Efficacy

Tumor immune escape refers to the ability of tumor cells to evade recognition and attack by the body's immune system through various mechanisms, allowing them to survive and proliferate in the body. While the body's natural and acquired immunity can resist brain tumor development, brain tumor cells can evade immune recognition and attack through various mechanisms. The occurrence and regression of brain tumors depend on the overall balance of these two opposing forces. Malignant brain tumors can evade the body's immune surveillance and proliferate rapidly in the body through a variety of mechanisms. In this section, we will discuss the mechanisms and characteristics of immune escape in brain tumors, using malignant glioma as an example, and examine the immunological characteristics of the tumor cells themselves, the altered host immune system, and the immune microenvironment.

(1) Glioma cells immune escape: Glioma cells possess unique immunological characteristics. On the one hand, these tumor cells are immunogenically weak or camouflage themselves through antigenic modulation. On the other hand, they express various immunomodulatory molecules and secrete cytokines that signal the host immune system to avoid attacking glioma cells. Tumor cells are derived from the host's own cells, and only a small fraction of abnormally expressed proteins are immunogenic. Additionally, these antigens are often obscured by certain molecules such as polysaccharides. During tumor progression, less immunogenic cells have a selective advantage in the growth process, a phenomenon known as immune selection. As a result, tumor cells become less and less immunogenic, causing the immune system to become "oblivious" to the tumor cells.

Most tumor cells have reduced or absent expression of major histocompatibility antigen-I (MHC-I) on their surface, which can lead to difficulties in T-cell recognition as it affects the formation of MHC-antigen peptide-TCR complexes. In a study of 88 surgical specimens, it was found that the expression of MHC class I molecules in gliomas was significantly downregulated and correlated with tumor grade. Furthermore, gliomas have low expression of MHC class II molecules and reduced expression of positive co-stimulatory molecules such as CD80 and CD86, while negative co-stimulatory molecules such as B7H1 and B7H4 are increased. This allows glioma cells to evade immune attack. Glioma cells also express Toll-like receptors, which promote tumor cell proliferation and inhibit apoptosis. Moreover, glioma cells express high levels of FasL (Fas ligand) but lack Fas expression, and since activated lymphocytes express both FasL and Fas, tumor cells can mediate apoptosis of immune effector cells through the FasL/Fas pathway, weakening the body's anti-tumor immune response. Glioma cells also express adhesion molecules such as CD28, ICAM1, IFA3, and VCAM1, which promote cell proliferation and participate in immune escape.

Glioma cells secrete or respond to various cytokines that can promote their own cell proliferation and negatively regulate host immunity. These cytokines include TGF-β, PGE2, IL-6, IL-10, CCL2, galectin-3, VEGF, and others. The negative immune factors induce the production of suppressive lymphocytes, such as suppressive monocytes and macrophages, inhibit T-cell differentiation, downregulate T cell adhesion and stimulatory molecules, and suppress CTL production by downregulating genes encoding perforin and granzyme B. TGF-β blocks DC maturation, inhibits T cell activation, and causes Treg amplification, while PGE2 downregulates MHC class II molecules and promotes Treg proliferation. CCL2 chemokine recruits Treg, and galectin-3, an adhesion molecule, induces T cell apoptosis by binding to HGG-expressed β-galactosides. These immune factors involve the common transcription factor STAT-3. Blocking STAT-3 with the small molecule inhibitor WP1066 or siRNA leads to a significant reduction in T-cell apoptosis and a consequent reduction in Treg.

Gliomas, like other malignant tumors, have a special group of cells known as GSCs, which possess a stronger ability to escape the immune system. They not only express negative immunomodulatory molecules and have low expression of MHC I molecules and NK cell activation ligands, but they can also tolerate Fas-mediated tumor cell apoptosis. These GSCs can evade the body's immune defense and become tumorigenic again, like entering a "no man's land," which makes anti-tumor immunity more challenging.

(2) Immune lymphocyte abnormalities: In addition to the immune properties of glioma cells themselves, there are also various abnormalities in the host immune system. Roszman and Brooks were the first to report lymphocyte abnormalities in brain tumor patients, including reduced ability of antigen-presenting cells (APCs) to present brain tumor antigens, as well as defective activation of T cells and NK cells.

Recently, there has been increased focus on microglia, Treg, and MDSC in the context of gliomas. Microglia are abundant in gliomas and contribute to the negative immune microenvironment in these tumors, potentially through the expression of the IDO gene. Treg cells are a subset of immune cells that negatively regulate immune function by suppressing the activation and function of CTLs and reducing cytokine production. Treg levels are significantly elevated in the tumor-infiltrating lymphocytes and peripheral blood mononuclear cells of glioma patients, particularly in HGG. Removal of Treg cells can significantly enhance the anti-tumor activity of CD4+ and CD8+ T cells. MDSCs were first identified in 1987 as a large subpopulation of suppressor cells in the peripheral blood and tumor-infiltrating tissues of patients with malignant glioma, characterized by the CD11b+Gr-1+ phenotype. MDSCs secrete high levels of TGF-β, NO, and arginase to promote T-cell apoptosis and inhibit T-cell proliferation, as well as promoting Treg production and downregulating the body's anti-tumor immunity. While the presence of MDSCs in glioma tissues has been confirmed, their specific classification and functional role require further investigation. It is important to note that the negative effects of these immune cells are not always consistent, as some studies have shown that the decreased T-cell response in tumor patients may be reversed in vitro with CD3 monoclonal antibody, CD28 monoclonal antibody, or IL-2, which can restore z-chain expression of CD3 molecules.

(3) Tumor immune microenvironment: Aside from the glioma cells' ability to evade immune detection, the tumor microenvironment also plays a crucial role in promoting tumor growth and infiltration while aiding glioma cells in evading the immune system. The tumor microenvironment is composed of tumor cells, stromal cells, and extracellular matrix. In gliomas, stromal cells mainly consist of microglia, fibroblasts, vascular endothelial cells, and immune/inflammatory cells. The tumor microenvironment serves as the primary "soil" for tumor cells, which, despite being hypoxic, acidic, and high-pressure, contain a significant number of growth factors, chemokines, protein hydrolases, and negative immunomodulatory factors. Tumor cells and the microenvironment have an interdependent relationship where they promote and antagonize each other through a "dialogue mechanism." Consequently, targeting the tumor microenvironment has become a promising area of research.

Some researchers have observed that gliomas formed by subcutaneous inoculation of GL261 cells are more sensitive to immunotherapy than those formed by intracranial injection. Moreover, intracranially formed gliomas have been found to have more Treg cells in the TILs. Pellegatta discovered that intra-tumoral injection of DC vaccine in gliomas was more effective than subcutaneous injection, indicating that the unique microenvironment of the central nervous system plays a crucial role in immunity. Microglia, which are believed to have antigen-presenting functions and are derived from the blood mononuclear macrophage system, require further exploration of their role in glioma. Fibroblasts are another group of stromal cells that have been infiltrated by malignant tumor cells and are involved in tumor immune escape by surrounding tumor cells and evading the host's anti-tumor immunity through the expression of fibroblast activation protein (FAP). Researchers used FAP knockout mice in a glioma model and found that anti-tumor immunity killed 80–90% of the tumor cells within 48 hours, while the control group had little to no protection from the tumor because of these stromal cells. Additionally, the tumor microenvironment induces vascular endothelial cells to provide tumors with camp. Research conducted at UCSF found that glioma cells with malignant EGFRv III mutations secrete IL-6, which causes surrounding tumor cells to express EGFRv III mutations and increase their malignancy. These cells are anchored to the stem cell niche by adhesion molecules, and their proliferation or differentiation depends on surrounding cytokines and activated signaling pathways. The tumor microenvironment is like a chronic inflammation with a large number of immunosuppressive cytokines, negative immunomodulatory cells, and inhibitory ligand-receptor responses, which allow for tumor growth, invasion, accelerated tumor progression, and immune escape despite the loss of immune surveillance.

Although several immunotherapy regimens for malignant brain tumors are available and have been proven to be safe and feasible, randomized controlled clinical trials are needed to confirm their effectiveness. Immunotherapy for brain tumors faces many difficulties, including a lack of specific antigens, tumor immune escape, and adverse effects of immunotherapy. While animal studies have produced promising results, human studies often fall short. Additionally, the immune system weakens with age, and the suppression of the immune system by chemotherapy and radiotherapy can significantly compromise immunotherapy. Glioma is a unique "cold" tumor in terms of immunity. Nonetheless, with the progress of immunomics, we believe that individualized immunotherapy for malignant brain tumors will eventually succeed in the near future.

Furthermore, utilizing immunological techniques for the diagnosis and treatment of gliomas, as well as utilizing tumor-infiltrating lymphocytes for staging or prognosis and leveraging immunological molecular characteristics of brain tumors for staging and treatment guidance, represents significant research directions for the future. It is important to recognize that immunotherapy serves as an adjuvant and complementary treatment. In clinical practice, biological immunology should be employed to eliminate and eradicate residual or spreading tumor cells at an early stage after the majority of the tumor has been removed through conventional surgery. This approach can improve and solidify the therapeutic effect and reduce the risk of recurrence. We eagerly await the continued progress of immunology and anticipate its future surprises in the field of anti-tumor immunotherapy.

10.5 Oncolytic Virus Would Offer a New Therapy for Gliomas

Oncolytic viruses (OV) are viruses that can selectively replicate and cause apoptosis of cancer cells while sparing normal tissues. OV therapy has been identified as a promising treatment strategy for gliomas, with more than 70 clinical trials reported to date. OVs can be classified into two main categories: natural viruses and genetically modified viruses. Both categories possess cytotoxicity and exhibit a preference for tumor tissues, enabling them to selectively infect tumor cells and replicate within them. This results in cytopathological effects, immune responses, and ultimately, the lysis of tumor cells.

Although the mechanisms of action of oncolytic viruses vary between categories, they share several common characteristics. These include:

Direct oncolytic action: After infecting target tumor cells, oncolytic viruses replicate heavily, leading to the rupture of these cells. The virus then reinfects neighboring cells to achieve continuous oncolytic action.

Activated and amplified immune responses: Oncolytic viruses induce immunogenic cell death, leading to the release of tumor-associated antigens and the infiltration of inflammatory cells. This stimulates anti-tumor immunity and enhances the sensitivity of tumor cells to cytokines. The antigen complex bound to MHC class I molecules on the surface of tumor cells can be recognized by CTLs, amplifying the anti-tumor immune effects.

Improved sensitivity to radiotherapy and chemotherapy: Studies have confirmed the synergistic effects of combining oncolytic viruses with radiotherapy or chemotherapy to improve therapy efficacy, although the specific mechanism requires further investigation.

Therapeutic expression of foreign genes: Oncolytic viruses can be genetically engineered to carry foreign anti-tumor genes. The expression of these genes can regulate cell function and achieve anti-tumor effects, such as the promotion of apoptosis of tumor cells by expressing the p53 gene.

Destruction of the tumor microenvironment: Oncolytic virus therapy promotes the formation of an inflammatory microenvironment around the tumor, including the release of pro-inflammatory cytokines, TLR ligands, innate immune cells, etc. The virus-induced tumor cell lysis and release of tumor antigens disrupt the immune homeostasis and internal structure of the tumor microenvironment.

Commonly used OVs include:

Herpes simplex virus-1 (HSV-1): Due to its natural neurotropism, genetically modified

HSV-1 was one of the first OVs tested for glioma therapy.

Adenovirus: The most commonly used adenovirus vector is derived from human Ad serotype 5 (AdHu5), but its clinical application is limited by the lack of receptors on glioma cells. In a Phase I clinical trial, modified adenovirus (Delta-24-RGD) was injected into the tumors of 25 patients with recurrent glioblastoma after surgeries or other treatments, resulting in a 20% survival rate of 3 years or longer. This is the first clinically relevant study reporting the direct oncolytic effects and anti-tumor immune response induced by OV.

Reovirus: Reovirus is a non-enveloped dsRNA virus that shows promising and efficient OV therapy due to its ability to restrict intratumor replication. Recent studies have shown a synergistic effect of combined reovirus therapy with conventional fractionated radiotherapy (FRT) and chemotherapy.

Measles virus (MV): Measles virus is an enveloped ssRNA virus. Genetically modified MV has been developed to target tumor-specific antigens, including EGFRvIII and high-affinity IL-13-binding transmembrane receptor alpha 2 (IL-13R2), in high-grade gliomas.

Poliovirus (PV): PV has been used to treat high-grade gliomas due to its specific affinity for CD155 (also known as poliovirus receptor or nectin-like molecule-5) and neurotropism in the brain. Genetic modification at the translational level to replace internal ribosome entry site (IRES) sequences in the PV genome with human rhinovirus 2 (HRV2) could enhance tumor specificity and minimize PV pathogenicity.

Delytact (teserpaturev/G47Δ) is the first OV product approved for the treatment of glioblastoma worldwide and has been currently approved in Japan. In a single-arm phase II trial, the genetically engineered HSV-1 OV showed a 1-year survival rate of 92.3%. MustangBio has initiated a Phase 1 clinical trial of a combination therapy for recurrent glioblastomas, consisting of MB-101 (an IL13Rα2-targeting CAR-T cell therapy) and MB-108 (an oncolytic therapy targeting C134). MB-109 is a combination of the two drugs aimed at improving the efficacy of MB-101 cell therapy by converting "cold" tumors into "hot" tumors. MB-108 oncolytic virus is designed to infect tumor cells and recruit endogenous CD8+ effector T cells, thereby reshaping the tumor microenvironment to allow for better infiltration, activation, and killing of tumor cells by MB-101 CAR-T cells. In preclinical studies, low doses of the combination therapy (MB-109) have been shown to be safe and effective in reducing tumor size. In preclinical studies, combination therapy has been shown to safely deliver low doses and lead to tumor shrinkage. A phase 1 clinical trial of DNX-2401 for the treatment of pediatric diffuse endogenous pontine gliomas was published in July 2022 in the New England Journal of Medicine, demonstrating the preliminary efficacy and safety of DNX-2401 in a single-center dose escalation study. Previous data from phase 2 trials of DNX-2401 in combination with pembrolizumab in recurrent glioblastomas showed a median overall survival of 12.5 months and a survival rate of 20.2% at 18 months. Many other OV trials are currently ongoing and highly anticipated.

Further Reading

Dams JL, Smothers J, Srinivasan R, et al. Big opportunities for small molecules immune-oncology. Nat Rev Drug Discov. 2015;14(9):603–22.

Elleg Atta S, Poliani PL, Stucchi E, et al. Intra-tumoral dendritic cells increase efficacy of peripheral vaccination by modulation of glioma microenvironment. Neuro Oncol. 2010;12(4):377–88.

Hua W, Yao Y, Chu Y, et al. The CD133+ tumor stem-like cell-associated antigen may elicit highly intense immune responses against human malignant glioma. J Neurooncol. 2011;105(2):149–57.

Jeon H, Vigdorovich V, Garrett-Thomson SC, et al. Structure and cancer immunotherapy of the B7 family member B7x. Cell Rep. 2014;9(3):1089–98.

Kalinina J, Peng J, Ritchie JC, et al. Proteomics of gliomas: initial biomarker discovery and evolution of technology. Neuro Oncol. 2011;13(9):926–42.

Kraman M, Bambrough PJ, Arnold JN, et al. Suppression of antitumor immunity by stromal cells expressing fibroblast activation protein-alpha. Science. 2010;330(6005):827–30.

Mahoney KM, Rennert PD, Freeman GJ. Combination cancer immunotherapy and new immunomodulatory targets. Nat Rev Drug Discov. 2015;14(8):561–84.

Mitchell DA, Batich KA, Gunn MD, et al. Tetanus toxoid and CCL3 improve dendritic cell vaccines in mice and glioblastoma patients. Nature. 2015;519(7543):366–9.

Nelson AL, Dhimolea E, Reichert JM. Development trends for human monoclonal antibody therapeutics. Nat Rev Drug Discov. 2010;9(10):767–74.

Okada H, Kalinski P, Ueda R, et al. Induction of CD8+ T-cell responses against novel glioma-associated antigen peptides and clinical activity by vaccinations with alpha-type 1 polarized dendritic cells and polyinosinic-polycytidylic acid stabilized by lysine and carboxymethylcellulose in patients with recurrent malignant glioma. J Clin Oncol. 2011;29(3):330–6.

Prins RM, Soto H, Konkankit V, et al. Gene expression profile correlates with T-cell infiltration and relative survival in glioblastoma patients vaccinated with dendritic cell immunotherapy. Clin Cancer Res. 2011;17(6):1603–15.

Sampson JH, Heimberger AB, Archer GE, et al. Immunologic escape after prolonged progression-free survival with epidermal growth factor receptor variant III peptide vaccination in patients with newly diagnosed glioblastoma. J Clin Oncol. 2010;28(31):4722–9.

Tang C, Wang XW, Li ZQ, et al. A systemic review of clinical trials on dendritic-cells based vaccine against malignant glioma. J Carcinogene Mutagene. 2015;6(2):1–7.

Wei H, Yu Y, Chu Y, et al. Phase I clinical trial study of human glioma stem cell-like antigen-sensitized dendritic cell vaccine. Chinese J Neurosurg. 2011;27(1):90–3.

11 Applications of Neuro-Oncology Multidisciplinary Team in Diagnosis and Treatment of Glioma

Jinsong Wu

11.1 MDT Is Essential in the Management of Glioma

The neuro-oncology multidisciplinary team (MDT) is a crucial organizational structure for providing evidence-based and personalized treatment for central nervous system neoplasms. MDTs are particularly effective for the treatment of complex gliomas that cannot be managed through routine therapy. The primary goal of MDT is to offer patient-centered, one-stop allied medical services that integrate the expertise of multidisciplinary teams in neuro-oncology. MDTs include core members such as neurosurgery, neuroimaging, neuropathology, radiation oncology, medical oncology, neurology, molecular pathology, hematology, endocrinology, neuropsychology, neurorehabilitation, clinical nursing, biospecimen banking, case room, hospice, and others, organized based on the disease stage and guided by critical clinical problems.

The neurosurgeon is the central figure in the neuro-oncology MDT, responsible for performing tumor resections, obtaining biological samples, directing patients for follow-up treatment, and following up on cases until the end of treatment. The MDT is headed by a medical secretary who organizes the team's regular meetings and coordinates patient management and referrals. The tumor board proposes the most suitable treatment plan for the patient's condition through multidisciplinary expert meetings, based on evidence-based medicine, and this plan is implemented by relevant disciplines individually or jointly. The MDT approach overcomes the limitations of single-specialty treatment, enhances communication and mutual understanding between different oncology specialties, ensures scientific implementation of tumor treatment, and embodies the standardization of tumor treatment. MDTs guide personalized precision medicine and promote the principle of evidence-based medicine in making medical decisions, making it an essential trend in the development of modern medicine. The concept of "MDT" was first introduced by the MD Anderson Cancer Center in the United States in the 1990s. Over the years, the MDT model has been widely adopted in many developed countries and regions, and the collaborative treatment mode of MDT is recommended in most cancer treatment guidelines. For example, the UK cancer treatment guidelines stipulate that all patients diagnosed with cancer must undergo relevant MDT consultation before receiving treatment, and the clinical decision of MDT must be adopted for the treatment of some malignant tumors. In the process of implementation, MDT quality standards have been gradually established, including regulations for team composition, clinician participation, meeting fre-

J. Wu (✉)
Department of Neurosurgery, Huashan Hospital, Fudan University, Shanghai, China

Y. Mao (ed.), *Progress in the Diagnosis and Treatment of Gliomas*, Experts' Perspectives on Medical Advances, https://doi.org/10.1007/978-981-99-0123-4_11

quency, and record-keeping of MDT decisions, ensuring the sustainable development of the MDT model. The MDT model for neuro-oncology was introduced later than other tumors, but it has also been highly emphasized and promoted in recent years.

MDT has become the preferred treatment model for most tumor treatments, according to the Guidelines for the Diagnosis and Treatment of Central Nervous System Tumors. Although the MDT model for neurological tumors started later in China, it has garnered significant attention in recent years, with many domestic hospitals establishing various forms of MDT models for neurological tumor diagnosis and treatment, achieving remarkable results. The third edition of the Chinese Guidelines for the Diagnosis and Treatment of CNS glioma specifically introduced the value of MDT in the diagnosis and treatment of neurological tumors. However, the implementation of MDT for neurological tumors has encountered several difficulties. Some relevant departments are not willing to transfer patients to other departments for consultation, as patients are used to receiving treatment within their own departments. In addition, the consultation process is often not standardized, and there may be incomplete records and summaries of opinions. There is also a lack of trust in the consultations received, and some departments may selectively record and implement them. Furthermore, there is a lack of practical problem-solving, and some departments may view it as a task or constraint. Finally, health economic cost accounting and other factors may also pose challenges. The main reason for these difficulties is a lack of understanding of MDT and the lack of unified standards to follow. Therefore, MDT has not yet become a routine treatment for tumors. The Huashan Glioma Center and the Neuro-Oncology MDT team were established by Huashan Hospital, Fudan University, in November 2011 under the advocacy and organization of Academician Zhou Liangfu. The team members consist of neurosurgeons, neuro-oncologists, neuro-imaging physicians, neuro-anesthesiologists, neuropathologists, radiologists, internal medicine physicians, digital medicine researchers, nursing staff, and technicians. To date, the team has discussed around 300 cases, effectively improving the therapeutic outcomes for brain tumor patients and achieving significant social benefits.

Based on the experience of the Neuro-Oncology MDT operation mode in Huashan Hospital, Fudan University, in recent years, we believe that several key issues are worth paying attention to. Firstly, it is essential to establish a standardized operation process, such as a centralized reporting system with a dedicated person in charge of contact, a unified reporting format, and clear requirements for the original data. A unified discussion system should also be implemented, with all participating members being experts with senior professional titles, a dedicated person to record the discussion, and the final results of the discussion as a guideline in principle. Additionally, implementing the medical treatment system and confirming the discussion plan is critical, informing the patient which doctor to seek. Secondly, it is important to pay attention to the important factors for the sustainability of the MDT, such as the interest of multidisciplinary physicians in the MDT, an equal voice in the discussion process, and encouragement and support from the hospital or higher levels. Thirdly, to ensure the objectivity and scientific nature of MDT treatment decisions, "let the data speak for itself" is crucial. Individualized precision medicine decisions should be guided by evidence-based raw data, not simply empirical medicine or the influence of traditional theoretical systems in the process of medical practice. Implementing medical decisions based on the principles of evidence-based medicine is essential to make medicine more scientific, standardized, and effective.

In the future, the development of MDT is likely to be combined with new mobile medical models, such as digital platforms like email groups and WeChat groups. This integration will break the limitations of time and space between multiple disciplines, but it will also put forward new requirements for medical security and patient privacy protection. Whether it's a traditional cancer conference, a joint clinic, or a new digital information exchange platform, MDT discussions should be conducted in a way that patients can understand, including treatment options, treatment timing, recommendations of the best-matched specialists, and taking into account cultural practices and educational background. The MDT should also support medical clinical research by collecting biospecimens and clinical information, documenting treatment decisions, and following up with the patient's prognosis with their informed consent. The MDT is also an important platform for medical education, where multidisciplinary discussions of difficult cases can enlighten young medical practitioners. Therefore, the MDT also serves as a continuing medical education function.

In conclusion, over the past few years, we have witnessed the MDT model becoming an inevitable trend for comprehensive and individualized treatment of neurological tumors. It is worth promoting the MDT model for neurological tumors throughout China. However, the MDT model for neurological tumors in China is not yet routine. Physicians' understanding of MDT is inadequate, and there are many problems in implementing trials in hospitals. Neuro-oncology professionals should actively seek policy support from national, regional, and hospital health management departments, collaborate collectively, learn from foreign advanced experiences, establish commendable organizational forms and institutional norms, and actively promote the development of neuro-oncology MDT.

Further Reading

European Partnership Action Against Cancer Consensus Group. Policy statement on multidisciplinary cancer care. Eur J Cancer. 2014;50(3):475–80.

Fennell ML, Das IP, Clauser S, et al. The organization of multidisciplinary care teams: modelling internal and external influences on cancer care quality. J Natl Cancer Inst Monogr. 2010;2010(40):72–80.

Nabors LB, Portnow J, Ammirati M, et al. Central nervous system cancers, version 1.2015. J Natl Compr Cancer Netw. 2015;13(10):1191–202.

National Institute for Health and Clinical Excellence. Guidance on cancer services: improving outcomes for people with brain and other CNS tumours. NICE: UK; 2006.

12 Clinical Trials on Glioma

Wei Hua and Xin Zhang

12.1 History of Clinical Trials

Glioma, the most common malignant tumor of the central nervous system, is also among the top 10 malignant tumors in terms of annual deaths. This devastating disease carries a poor prognosis, high disability rate, and a substantial economic burden on society and families. Despite these challenges, significant advancements have been made in the diagnosis and treatment of glioma. Previously, the surgical goal was focused on "saving lives," but now the aim is to "protect neurological function" while treating the tumor. The classification of gliomas has also evolved from traditional histomorphological classification to a more comprehensive approach that includes molecular pathology and histomorphology. Molecular biomarkers such as IDH mutation, H3K27M mutation, and 1p/19q co-deletion have been introduced in the NCCN CNS tumor guideline, revolutionizing the diagnosis, treatment, and prognosis of glioma and ushering it into the era of molecular typing. As the field of "precision medicine" continues to advance, clinical trials will play a critical role in glioma research.

The history of medicine is widely believed to have originated from the ancient empirical phase (2000 BC to sixteenth century AD), during which people accumulated vast amounts of traditional medical knowledge and experience. This knowledge was heavily influenced by religious and philosophical ideas from different regions and periods, ultimately leading to the development of a new system of medicine. Throughout this period, a number of classical books were produced, including the ancient Babylonian "Diagnostic Manual," the Hebrew "Pentateuch," the Egyptian "Papyrus," the Indian "Pharmacopoeia," and "Surgery," the Roman "Canon of Medicine," and the Chinese "The Yellow Emperor's Classic of Internal Medicine" and "The Compendium of Materia Medica."

The sixteenth-century Renaissance marked the beginning of a medical revolution, which gained momentum as knowledge of anatomy and physiology accumulated. With the development of technology and life science, modern medicine came into its own. Clinical trials have been conducted for nearly 300 years, with the first known clinical trial occurring in Britain in the eighteenth century. At the time, scurvy was a significant health problem for the British Navy due to vitamin C deficiency. In 1747, James Lind, a naval physician, designed the first controlled clinical trial to compare six different treatments for scurvy. His study concluded that citrus and lemon were the most effective in treating the disease. The paper reporting the results of this landmark study was published in 1753 and is considered to be the first controlled clinical trial. James Lind is

W. Hua · X. Zhang (✉)
Department of Neurosurgery, Huashan Hospital, Fudan University, Shanghai, China

Y. Mao (ed.), *Progress in the Diagnosis and Treatment of Gliomas*, Experts' Perspectives on Medical Advances, https://doi.org/10.1007/978-981-99-0123-4_12

Table 12.1 Clinical trial staging

Phase of the trial	Trial design	Purpose of the trial	Cases of enrollment included
Phase I	Open-label, dose escalating	Determining the maximal tolerated dose. Obtaining pharmacokinetic data	Usually, 20 ~ 30
Phase II	Randomized, double-blind, controlled trial	Determining the efficacy in a specific population	No less than 100
Phase III	Randomized, double-blind, positive controlled	Determining the safety and efficacy in a larger population	No less than 300
Phase IV	Open-label, no control group	Efficacy, adverse effects	Greater than 2000
EAP clinical trials	Not required	Providing new treatments for patients who are not suitable for clinical trials	Not required

widely recognized as one of the pioneers in the development of controlled clinical trials.

The first randomized controlled trial that is widely accepted in medical research was conducted by Geoffrey Marshall in 1948 and published in the British Medical Journal. This trial, which tested the efficacy of streptomycin in the treatment of tuberculosis, was conducted at multiple centers across the UK and provided conclusive evidence that streptomycin was effective in treating the disease. Since the publication of Marshall's trial, clinical trials have become more widespread around the world and are now an essential part of the process of introducing new drugs and treatments into clinical practice.

The development of clinical trials has not been without challenges, as the misuse or lack of safety assessment of subjects by some investigators has led to catastrophic consequences, such as the "thalidomide tragedy." In response to these incidents, the Declaration of Helsinki was adopted by the 18th World Medical Association General Assembly in Finland in June 1964, emphasizing the primary responsibility of physicians to promote and safeguard the health, well-being, and rights of patients. Furthermore, Good Clinical Practice (GCP) guidelines were introduced in many countries to regulate the conduct of clinical trials and ensure that they are conducted in a safe and ethical manner. GCP provides a framework for designing, conducting, and reporting clinical trials that ensures the rights, safety, and well-being of trial participants are protected. It also provides guidelines for data management and quality assurance to ensure that the results of the trial are reliable and accurate.

12.2 Concepts and Guidelines for Clinical Trials

What is a clinical trial? According to the Code of Quality Management for Drug Clinical Trials issued by the former China Food and Drug Administration (CFDA), a clinical trial is a systematic study of a drug or intervention in humans (either patients or healthy volunteers) to evaluate the drug's efficacy, safety, and other pharmacological properties, such as absorption, distribution, metabolism, and excretion. This includes a wide range of interventions, such as clinical drugs, radiotherapy, viral therapy, and distinct surgical approaches. Well-designed and scientifically conducted clinical trials are crucial in advancing human health and discovering new therapeutic drugs and methods, as they offer a fast and safe means of assessing new treatments.

Clinical trials are typically divided into several phases, including Phase I, II, III, and IV, as well as EAP clinical trials (Table 12.1). Phase I clinical trials involve initial evaluations of clinical pharmacology, human safety, and pharmacokinetics to determine the maximum tolerated dose and obtain pharmacokinetic data of the new drug. These trials are usually open-label, dose-escalating studies that include 20–30 healthy subjects or patients, and CFDA approval must be obtained before the trial begins. Phase II clinical trials are designed to initially evaluate the therapeutic effect and safety of the drug in patients with the indication. They typically use blinded randomized controlled trials, often using double-blind randomized parallel controlled trials, and usually include no fewer than 100 patients. Phase III clinical trials are the verification phase of therapeutic effects, which aim to further confirm the therapeutic effect and safety of the drug in patients with the target indication, evaluate the benefit-risk relationship, and provide a sufficient basis for the review of the drug registration application. These trials have the same design requirements as phase II blinded randomized controlled trials but may use blinded or unblinded randomized controlled open-label trials. Phase III clinical trials usually include no fewer than 300 patients, and once a drug successfully completes phase III, it can be officially marketed. Phase IV clinical trials are applied studies that are conducted after a new drug has been marketed. The goal is to investigate the efficacy and adverse effects of the drug under wider application, evaluate the benefit-risk relationship in general or special populations, and improve the dosing regimen. These trials are typically open-label without a control group, and small sample randomized controls are also possible. According to CFDA regulations, Phase IV trials require at least 2000 subjects.

An Expanded Access Program (EAP) clinical trial is a type of clinical trial conducted by a pharmaceutical company that provides patients with serious medical conditions, who are not suitable for participation in controlled clinical trials, the opportunity to receive treatment with a new investigational drug under certain conditions. Patients may be ineligible to participate in controlled clinical trials due to their health status, age, or other factors that would prevent them from being enrolled. For example, a patient may live too far from a clinical research center. However, these patients may still benefit from the new drug. The FDA allows pharmaceutical companies to provide access to the new drug under certain conditions, through an "expanded pathway," in order to benefit these patients.

Clinical trials play a crucial role in drug development, but it is essential to design and conduct them in strict compliance with Chinese laws, regulations, and international standards. The regulations cover every aspect of the trial, from design and subject recruitment to record-keeping and analysis of results. The key laws and regulations include the "Drug Administration Law of the People's Republic of China," "Regulations for the Implementation of the Drug Administration Law of the People's Republic of China," "Measures for the Administration of Drug Registration," "Code of Practice for the Quality Management of Non-Clinical Drug Research," "Code of Practice for the Quality Management of Clinical Drug Trials," "Measures for Handling Violations in Drug Research and Registration Application," "Interim Provisions for Drug Research Experiment Records," "Measures for the Administration of Reporting and Monitoring of Adverse Drug Reactions," and "Declaration of Helsinki," among others. Compliance with these regulations is essential to ensure the safety of trial participants and the validity of trial results.

12.3 The Conduct of Clinical Trials in Glioma

The drug treatment of glioma involves a variety of methods, such as alkylating agent-based chemotherapy, targeted therapy, and immunotherapy. However, before these drugs can be used in clinical practice, they must first undergo rigorous validation in the preclinical stage, including in vitro tests and animal models, and then clinical trials at various stages. Unfortunately, only a small fraction of these drugs (less than 1%) has been found to be safe and effective for use in the clinical setting. Glioma is the most common malignant tumor in the central nervous system, posing a significant challenge for neuro-oncologists. Given the heterogeneity of glioma and the development of drug resistance due to the activation of the blood-brain barrier and other pathways, the treatment of glioma patients remains challenging.

(1) Trial design: Clinical trials for glioma must be carefully designed to ensure the safety and efficacy of the drugs being tested. The trial design process should consider several factors, including whether to randomize, whether to include a control group, the selection of a control group, and whether to use a blinded method. When designing clinical trials for glioma drug therapy, researchers should consider factors such as whether to use a single agent, drug combination, or combination with radiotherapy, whether the trial is for primary or recurrent glioma, and the age and location of patients with glioma. Additionally, clinical trials should also be conducted to evaluate surgical treatments for glioma.

(2) Enrollment requirements: In clinical trials for glioma, subjects must meet certain requirements. For newly diagnosed glioma trials, screening should be completed within a short period after surgery. For recurrent glioma trials, measurable lesions on imaging are generally required. Other requirements include pathology, age, lesion characteristics, physical and functional status scores (such as ECOG or KPS), and routine blood and biochemistry tests. A washout period is generally required before the start of the clinical trial for recurrent glioma trials to exclude the effects of the previous treatment. Since patients with recurrent glioma often have neurological dysfunction, the KPS or ECOG scores may need to be adjusted, or else it may cause difficulties in enrollment.

(3) Imaging assessment [response assessment in neuro-oncology (RANO), modified RANO]: The size of the glioma lesion during the screening stage is determined based on the imaging presentation, usually cranial enhanced MRI, and serves as the baseline for evaluation. Follow-up MRIs are then performed as required by the protocol to assess whether the lesion has progressive disease (PD), stable disease (SD), partial response (PR), or complete response (CR). The RANO criteria proposed by Wen et al. (Table 12.2) is currently the most widely used imaging assessment method in glioma clinical trials. It evaluates T1 enhancement, T2 FLAIR, new lesion appearance, use of corticosteroids, and clinical presentation. Although the RANO criteria are widely accepted, modifications have been made to address its shortcomings.

(4) Choosing the endpoint of the trial: In traditional clinical trials, overall survival (OS), progression-free survival (PFS), and overall response rate (ORR) are commonly used as endpoints. High-grade glioma (HGG) trials often use OS and PFS as endpoints, while low-grade glioma (LGG) trials may use PFS or annual survival rate as the endpoint, since LGG has a better prognosis compared to HGG.

Table 12.2 RANO standards

Project	Complete remission (CR)	Partial relief (PR)	Stable (SD)	Progress (PD)
T+ enhancement	Not yet seen	Reduce by ≥50%	Changes between −50 and +25%	Increase by ≥25%*
T2/FLAIR	Stable or decreasing	Stable or decreasing	Stable or decreasing	Increase*
Newly added lesions	Not yet seen	Not yet seen	Not yet seen	Visible*
Corticosteroid application	Need not	Stable or decreasing	Stable or decreasing	Not as a standard
Clinical manifestation	Stable or improved	Stable or improved	Stable or improved	Deteriorate*
Conditions required for judgment criteria	All of the above	All of the above	All of the above	Any of the above

Note: Any item containing * is considered progress, not as a standard. If there is no clinical deterioration, an increase in corticosteroid dosage alone cannot determine progression

(5) IRB and clinical trial registration: Before the start of a clinical trial, it must pass the review of the Ethics Committee and be conducted in strict compliance with the requirements of GCP. Additionally, the trial must be registered with relevant organizations, such as the Clinical Trials website (https://clinicaltrials.gov/) and the corresponding website in China. The trial status must be updated regularly on these websites to ensure transparency and accessibility of trial information to the public.

12.4 Current Status of Clinical Trials in Glioma

As of January 2018, a total of 1934 glioma clinical trials were actively recruiting globally on the Clinical Trials website, with 1329 trials being conducted in the US and 64 trials in China. Among these trials, 41.10% were in phase I, 50.74% were in phase II, 7.6% were in phase III, and 0.57% were in phase IV. Over the years, there has been a gradual increase in the number of randomized controlled trials (RCTs) in neurosurgery, with significant improvements in the design of neurosurgical intervention RCTs in several aspects. As a result, many of these trials are now considered classic clinical trials.

(1) Clinical trials of classic chemotherapeutic agents: The most notable example is the phase III clinical trial conducted by Stupp et al. in 2005, which demonstrated the effectiveness of post-surgical temozolomide in combination with radiotherapy in the treatment of glioblastoma, and extended the median survival of glioblastoma to 14.6 months, a significant milestone in glioma clinical research. Many new interventions have been added to the standard Stupp regimen, and the number of clinical trials for glioma has increased rapidly. For instance, in 2015, The Journal of the American Medical Association reported that combining TTF with temozolomide significantly improved PFS and OS in GBM patients compared to temozolomide alone, based on a study of 695 GBM patients. Apart from clinical trials for GBM, clinical trials for LGG have also been conducted. The scope and complexity of these trials are greater due to the longer survival of LGG patients. For example, a clinical trial that combined the PCV regimen (procarbazine + lomustine + vincristine) with radiotherapy enrolled 251 subjects between 1998 and 2002, with a median follow-up of 11.9 years. The results of this trial indicated that the OS and PFS of the combined therapy group were significantly prolonged for WHO grade II glioma patients. The final results were published in the New England Journal of Medicine in 2016.

(2) Clinical trials of targeted therapies: Clinical trials can yield both successful and unsuccessful outcomes. Avastin, a VEGFA monoclonal antibody, has shown efficacy in treating advanced colon, lung, and kidney cancers. Given its antiangiogenic properties, Avastin was expected to be effective in treating gliomas, which are highly vascularized tumors. However, a study published in the Journal of Clinical Oncology in 2011 reported that combining bevacizumab with the Stupp regimen did not significantly prolong overall survival (OS) or progression-free survival (PFS) in 70 GBM cases compared to using the Stupp regimen alone.

(3) Immunotherapy clinical trials: In recent years, there has been a growing interest in immunotherapy, and various vaccines targeting IDH1 mutation and H3.3K27M are currently in phase I clinical trials for glioma. The effectiveness of immunotherapy in improving the prognosis of glioma patients is yet to be established through further phase II and III clinical trials. The latest breakthrough in glioma treatment is viral transgenesis, where oncolytic viruses are genetically modified to target and eliminate tumor cells. Currently, genetically modified adenovirus DNX-2401 and second-generation oncolytic herpes simplex virus M032 are undergoing phase I clinical trials.

As our understanding of diseases continues to advance, innovative therapeutic approaches are emerging and gaining momentum. One such approach is chimeric antigen receptor-modified T cells (CAR-T), an immunotherapy that has demonstrated promising results in treating melanoma, leukemia, and neuroblastoma. In the case of glioma, several clinical trials are currently underway, and there is one noteworthy instance reported in The New England Journal of Medicine: a 50-year-old male with right temporal lobe glioblastoma (GBM) who relapsed 6 months after undergoing the standard Stupp regimen. He received treatment with CAR-T therapy targeting IL13 Rα2, which resulted in a significant reduction in the tumor size in the skull and spinal cord, and a progression-free survival (PFS) of 7.5 months. Although multiple tumor relapses occurred in distal sites eventually, this case highlights the potential of CAR-T therapy in treating GBM.

(4) Other clinical trials: Proton beam therapy is an advanced form of radiation treatment that offers greater specificity in targeting tumors than conventional radiotherapy that uses X-rays. The lack of specificity is a major challenge associated with traditional radiotherapy. Proton beam therapy, on the other hand, has the ability to deliver higher doses of radiation to tumors while minimizing exposure to surrounding healthy tissues.

In 1991, the Loma Linda University Medical Center (LLUMC) made history by introducing the first proton device for medical use, marking a significant milestone in the development of proton therapy. Unlike traditional radiotherapy that uses X-rays, medical protons are obtained from ionizing hydrogen (H2) into protons (H) and accelerating them to near the speed of light using a synchrotron or cyclotron for therapeutic purposes. The unique dose distribution pattern of protons generates what is known as the Bragg peak. By precisely placing the lesion at the peak, a high therapeutic gain ratio can be achieved with a single field of the proton beam, setting protons apart from X-rays and gamma-ray light.

Subs have a distinct advantage in radiation therapy and have been utilized in Phase II trials for gliomas. The Department of Neurosurgery at Huashan Hospital, Fudan University, is currently collaborating with the Shanghai Proton Heavy Ion Hospital to conduct a clinical trial on adaptive radiation treatment of intracranial tumors using multimodal imaging guidance. The study plans to recruit 42 subjects to participate.

12.5 Difficulties and Prospects for Conducting Clinical Trials in Glioma

(1) Problems and Difficulties

Despite a significant increase in the number of clinical trials conducted for gliomas, only a few have been successful. Clinical trials demand substantial investments of time and money by investigators and sponsors, yet only a small fraction of them prove effective in the clinic. Many of the 70 trials conducted since the first RCT in the 1940s have used the same protocols, resulting in high costs with limited efficiency. Traditional clinical trials have significantly hindered the development of tumor treatments.

The heterogeneity of gliomas is partly responsible for the difficulty in finding a single cure that works for all glioma patients. Despite the selection of small molecular compounds with good blood-brain barrier permeability, tumor resistance can still develop, and once a tumor recurs, the progression is rapid. Furthermore, with a relatively low incidence rate and dispersed neurological centers, conducting large-scale clinical trials poses a significant challenge. Regular follow-up care in domestic medical centers has only recently begun. Even in developed countries, only 21% of patients are aware of or participate in clinical trials.

In China, there are additional obstacles such as slow approval of new drugs and a high dependence on generic drugs with a lack of innovative treatments.

(2) Proposed Adaptive Clinical Trials

In order to enhance the effectiveness of clinical trials, particularly for targeted tumor drugs, and provide more individualized treatment for tumor patients, experts have suggested the use of adaptive clinical trials. Due to difficulties in enrolling certain rare targets in precision therapy, adaptive trials have been proposed as a potential solution. The concept of adaptive trials aims to address multiple issues in the shortest amount of time possible. It features a master protocol, which includes one or more treatment protocols for one or more diseases or targets, allowing for the resolution of various clinical problems. The three main types of adaptive clinical trials are basket trials, umbrella trials, and platform trials.

(a) A basket trial focuses on the same target across different diseases and subjects. For instance, the B2225 clinical trial evaluated the efficacy of imatinib on a variety of 40 tumors.
(b) An umbrella trial involves the use of different targeted therapies for individuals with the same or specific diseases based on multiple targets. For instance, the NCI-MATCH clinical trials for advanced solid tumors, lymphoma, and myeloma employ this approach.
(c) Platform trials can be viewed as an evolution and expansion of umbrella trials, which allow investigators to add drugs to a treatment platform at their discretion. Throughout the trial, the investigator can stop a drug in a group and replace it with a new drug in the platform. If a drug proves effective, it can be promoted to become the standard treatment for that group. Prominent examples of platform trials include the I-SPY 2 trial for breast cancer and the lung-MAP trial for lung cancer.

The advantage of this trial protocol is that it allows for the evaluation of safety and efficacy of targeted drugs by analyzing common characteristics among different types of tumor subjects or different targets in the same subject. This approach is faster and more effective than traditional single-drug clinical trials in screening potentially effective targeted drugs.

The GBM adaptive global clinical trial in 2015 introduced a new clinical trial model for glioma researchers: a learning adaptive multicenter clinical trial. This trial model groups subjects with different targets and employs sequential or combined treatment with multiple drugs, while also collecting tumor specimens and sequencing data for future studies. This approach maximizes resources and efficiency in the face of limited subject availability.

Furthermore, recent revisions to the national new drug access system are expected to expedite the review process for new drugs. Nevertheless, it remains essential to enhance patient awareness of clinical trials and promote patient engagement in such trials.

Further Reading

Berry DA. The brave new world of clinical cancer research: adaptive biomarker-driven trials integrating clinical practice with clinical research. Mol Oncol. 2015;9(5):951–9.

Brown CE, Alizadeh D, Starr R, et al. Regression of glioblastoma after chimeric antigen receptor T-cell therapy. N Engl J Med. 2016;375(26):2561–9.

Buckner JC, Shaw EG, Pugh SL, et al. Radiation plus Procarbazine, CCNU, and vincristine in low-grade glioma. N Engl J Med. 2016;374(14):1344–55.

Ellingson BM, Wen PY, Cloughesy TF. Modified criteria for radiographic response assessment in glioblastoma clinical trials. Neurotherapeutics. 2017;14(2):307–20.

Lai A, Tran A, Nghiemphu PL, et al. Phase II study of bevacizumab plus temozolomide during and after radiation therapy for patients with newly diagnosed glioblastoma multiforme. J Clin Oncol. 2011;29(2):142–8.

Louis DN, Perry A, Reifenberger G, et al. The 2016 World Health Organization classification of tumors of the central nervous system: a summary. Acta Neuropathol. 2016;131(6):803–20.

Stupp R, Mason WP, Van Den Bent MJ, et al. Radiotherapy plus concomitant and adjuvant temozolomide for glioblastoma. N Engl J Med. 2005;352(10):987–96.

Stupp R, Taillibert S, Kanner AA, et al. Maintenance therapy with tumor-treating fields plus temozolomide vs temozolomide alone for glioblastoma: a randomized clinical trial. JAMA. 2015;314(23):2535–43.

Wen PY, MacDonald DR, Reardon DA, et al. Updated response assessment criteria for high-grade gliomas: response assessment in neuro-oncology working group. J Clin Oncol. 2010;28(11):1963–72.

Woodcock J, Lavange LM. Master protocols to study multiple therapies, multiple diseases, or both. N Engl J Med. 2017;377(1):62–70.

Physiotherapy for Glioma

13

Jinsen Zhang and Wei Hua

Physical therapy for tumors involves utilizing natural or artificial physical energy to prevent and treat tumors. This type of therapy has a long history of being used for tumor prevention and rehabilitation. However, physical therapy for brain tumors can be limited due to the physical barriers of the skull bone and the blood-brain barrier. Nevertheless, some methods have been developed to overcome these physical barriers, which can be used as complementary options or to enhance sensitivity to treatment.

Common methods used in glioma treatment include photodynamic therapy (PDT), laser interstitial thermal therapy (LITT), and soundynamic therapy (SDT). One popular method is tumor treating fields (TTFields). This chapter will primarily focus on TTFields as an example for discussing physiotherapy for glioma.

TTFields are a cancer treatment that uses low-intensity, intermediate-frequency electric fields to interrupt cell division and kill tumor cells. Studies have shown that TTFields can prolong the survival of patients with glioblastoma (GBM). The FDA approved TTFields for the treatment of recurrent GBM in 2011 and newly diagnosed GBM in 2015. According to the Central Nervous System Tumor Guidelines (2017), TTFields can be applied to GBM patients with a Karnofsky Performance Status (KPS) score of ≥60, regardless of MGMT promoter methylation status, and can be combined with temozolomide after standard concurrent radio-chemotherapy for patients ≤70 years old. Patients aged over 70 years who receive non-hyperfractionated radiotherapy and opt for standard concurrent radio-chemotherapy may also benefit from combined TTFields treatment.

13.1 How TTFields Works

(1) Overview

TTFields can potentially disrupt the normal mitotic process by influencing critical molecules or organelles that are charged during mitosis, leading to tumor suppression. This disruption occurs through two basic physical principles: dipole alignment and dielectric electrophoresis. In response to a uniform alternating electric field, charged molecules undergo continuous oscillations, causing the separation of positive and negative charges within the molecule and aligning themselves in parallel to the direction of the electric force vector. During mitosis and cytoplasmic division, key macromolecules and organelles are hyperpolarized, allowing charged structures at each stage of cell division to align precisely. However, the applied local electric field can disturb the random motions of these structures, leading to

J. Zhang · W. Hua (✉)
Department of Neurosurgery, Huashan Hospital, Fudan University, Shanghai, China

Y. Mao (ed.), *Progress in the Diagnosis and Treatment of Gliomas*, Experts' Perspectives on Medical Advances, https://doi.org/10.1007/978-981-99-0123-4_13

disruption of cell division and potential tumor suppression.

TTFields can disrupt the normal movement of microtubule subunits in the cytoplasm during metaphase, leading to abnormal microtubule assembly in the spindle and resulting in asymmetric chromatin segregation. During normal cell division, septin 2/6/7 aggregates are recruited to the midline portion of the spindle at a later stage, and the oval groove narrows due to the action of parallel distributed septin fibers, with the division axis aligned parallel to the direction of the applied alternating electric field. However, TTFields can interfere with this process and inhibit septin formation by disrupting the ability of individual aggregates to bind to each other. In the absence of normal cytosolic protein function, cell contraction cannot be confined to the equatorial midline, leading to violent contraction of the cell membrane and abnormal mitotic exits in the late phase, eventually resulting in cytoplasmic blistering and membrane rupture. Moreover, microtubule proteins have a high electric dipole moment, and the effect of TTFields on microtubules may be more significant due to the rapid dynamic process of microtubule assembly and dissociation. Consequently, TTFields can cause asymmetric chromatin segregation, mitotic inhibition, or delayed division in dividing cells, leading to uneven distribution of chromosomes in daughter cells and ultimately resulting in cellular stress. Tumor cells under stress induced by TTFields can trigger immune response effects in the host.

TTFields exhibit both direct and indirect antitumor mechanisms, and their effectiveness is enhanced when the host's immune system is simultaneously activated. Immunofluorescence microscopy can reveal the abnormal structure of tumor cells treated with TTFields. The frequency of the alternating electric field impacts these cellular phenomena, with an effective range of 100–300 kHz and an optimal frequency of 200 kHz. This optimal frequency is related to cell size, which may explain the variation in optimal frequencies observed in mesothelioma cell lines (NCI-H2052 and MSTO-211H), lung adenocarcinoma cells (A549 and H1299), breast adenocarcinoma, and GBM.

(2) Factors Affecting the Treatment of TTFields

TTFields induce abnormal tumor cell division and are influenced by various physical factors, including the frequency and intensity of the electric field. Wenger et al. conducted computational modeling of intracellular TTFields and found that frequencies below 10 kHz failed to penetrate the cell membrane, while the electric field at 200 kHz achieved the greatest penetration effect when concentrated in the cellular dynamical furrow. Additionally, the effect of the applied electric field is directional, with maximum field strength obtained when dividing cells are oriented parallel to the applied electric field (at an angle 0), and minimum strength obtained when cells are oriented perpendicular to the electric field (at an angle 90). Partial effects are observed between 0° and 90°, with field strength decreasing as cells are oriented from 0° to 90°. Moreover, the antitumor effect of TTFields is dependent on intensity and time, with stronger field strengths resulting in greater inhibition of tumor cell line proliferation and longer durations of TTFields leading to more significant inhibition of proliferation activity in tumor cell lines.

During TTFields treatment, the distribution of the electric field is not uniform and is influenced by factors such as the geometry of the organ being treated, the distance of the energy converter, and the tissue's dielectric properties. Additionally, the electric field does not decay with distance from the electrodes and does not exhibit a half-life, allowing for continuous application during treatment, which is one of the benefits of TTFields therapy.

(3) Other Mechanisms of TTFields

TTFields have been found to interrupt not only cell division but also DNA repair mechanisms. Analysis of gene expression in lung cancer cell lines treated with TTFields for 72 h showed that the BRCA1 pathway was more strongly inhibited compared to the control group. This effect was more pronounced in responding cell lines such as H57 and H4006 than in non-responding cell lines like A549 and H1299. Furthermore, flow cytometric analysis showed that the responding cell lines had higher levels of DNA double-strand breaks and sub-G1 phase cells, suggesting that TTFields induced a higher rate of apoptosis by interrupting the DNA repair mechanism. The formation of R-Loop structures associated with DNA replication stress was also observed after TTFields treatment, indicating an increase in intracellular DNA replication stress. This makes cells more susceptible to cytocidal effects from DNA-damaging agents, such as PARP inhibitors. This mechanism of action is independent and simultaneous with the mitogenic effect of TTFields.

TTFields may also induce an immune response in the host, indirectly inhibiting tumor cell growth. TTFields disrupt the division process of cells, causing them to release cellular stress signals such as calreticulin and HMGB1. Tali Voloshin et al. discovered that the combination of TTFields and anti-PD-1 treatment induced changes in the tumor microenvironment and promoted the phagocytosis of TTFields-treated cells by bone marrow-derived dendritic cells. Conversely, the control group did not display similar effects. Furthermore, in a study conducted by the same group, Lewis lung cancer cells were injected directly into the lungs of male C57Bl/6 mice, and TTFields were applied to the lungs of the mice for 7 days while anti-PD-1 drugs were administered intraperitoneally. Results showed a significant decrease in tumor volume and an increase in leukocytes (CD45+) in the group receiving the combination of TTFields and anti-PD-1 treatment.

Kirson et al. conducted an experiment where they injected highly metastatic VX-2 tumors in the kidneys of rabbits and treated them with TTFields. The results showed a significant reduction in the number of distant lung metastases compared to the sham control group. This suggests that TTFields may have a potential immunomodulatory effect and induce immunogenic cell death, ultimately leading to tumor elimination.

13.2 Efficacy of TTFields-TMZ Combination Therapy in Patients with Primary GBM

To evaluate the efficacy of TTFields-TMZ combination therapy, Stuppa et al. conducted a randomized clinical trial involving 210 patients receiving TTFields in combination with TMZ and 105 patients receiving TMZ alone. The results showed that the median PFS was 7.1 months (95% CI: 5.9–8.2 months) in the combination group, which was significantly longer than the 4 months (95% CI: 3.3–5.2 months) observed in the TMZ group. Furthermore, the combination therapy group had a longer overall survival (OS) of 20.5 months (95% CI: 16.7–25.0 months), compared to only 15.6 months (95% CI: 13.3–19.1 months) in the TMZ group.

The subsequent trial yielded similar results, with 466 patients randomly assigned to the TTFields-TMZ combination therapy group and 229 patients to the TMZ-only group. The median PFS for patients in the TTFields-TMZ combination group was 6.7 months, compared to 4.0 months in the TMZ-only group (HR = 0.63, 95% CI: 0.52–0.67). The 6-month PFS rates were 56% and 37% (95% CI: 0.51–0.61) in the TTFields-TMZ and TMZ-only groups, respectively. The TTFields-TMZ group also had a longer OS of 20.9 months compared to 16.0 months in the TMZ-only group (HR = 0.63, 95% CI: 0.53–0.76). The proportion of patients who survived for more than 2 years after enrollment was higher in the TTFields-TMZ group (43%) than in the TMZ-only group (29%). Moreover, patients who complied well with the treatment had the greatest survival benefit.

No unanticipated adverse effects were observed during the application of TTFields.

Grade 3 or 4 side effects were similar between the two groups, mainly involving blood, gastrointestinal disturbances, and cramps. Scalp reactions were only observed in the TTFields group. There was no significant increase in systemic toxic effects in patients with newly diagnosed GBM treated with TTFields-TMZ compared to TMZ treatment alone. However, a higher incidence of local dermal problems was observed in patients treated with TTFields-TMZ. Mild to moderate skin irritation was observed in 43% of patients treated with TTFields-TMZ, and severe skin reactions (grade 3) were observed in 2% of patients. The incidence of mild anxiety, confusion, insomnia, and headache was higher in TTFields-TMZ-treated patients and occurred mainly at the beginning of treatment. Seizure rates were almost identical in the two groups. Because TTFields were applied only to the head, no increase in systemic adverse effects or seizure rates or neurological adverse effects was observed. A total of 12 patients died from causes unrelated to adjuvant therapy.

This study demonstrated that TTFields therapy as an adjuvant to TMZ improved survival in patients with primary GBM compared to TMZ therapy alone, and prolonged PFS. The results were consistent with those of other GBM clinical trials. However, it is important to note that patients in this trial were randomized only at the end of radiotherapy, and the first cycle of maintenance TMZ therapy was started at the time of grouping, thus excluding patients with early tumor progression during radiotherapy. Furthermore, while most GBM trials report survival from the date of initial diagnosis or study enrollment in radiotherapy, this trial reported survival from the time of randomization, which resulted in a 3-month increase in survival time that has significant clinical implications.

One limitation of this study was that patients were enrolled after completing radiotherapy, resulting in a difference in the timing of standard TMZ and radiotherapy treatment. Patients with early progression during radiotherapy could not be included in the randomization, which excluded those with a poor prognosis. Due to patient and caregiver burden and the need to shave hair and apply electrode sheets, a placebo or sham control was neither feasible nor appropriate. The trial design was similar to the study evaluating radiotherapy. Post-analysis revealed that patients over the age of 65 had shorter survival than those under 65, but both groups still had significantly higher survival rates. Additionally, while treatment with TTFields-TMZ was associated with longer survival, patients with tumors lacking MGMT promoter methylation had significantly shorter survival compared to those with MGMT promoter methylation.

13.3 TTFields for the Treatment of Recurrent Glioblastoma

(1) Early Clinical Trials

In 2007, Kirson et al. conducted a clinical trial using TTFields to treat recurrent glioma in 10 patients. The study demonstrated promising results, with a median PFS of 26.1 weeks and a 6-month PFS of 50%. At the end of the study, two patients were still progression-free. The median OS was 62.2 weeks, which was much longer than previous studies and confirmed the efficacy of TTFields. Additionally, the study found that nerve and muscle excitation were not significantly disturbed by TTFields treatment for alternating fields greater than 10 kHz due to the parallel resistor-capacitor nature of the cell membrane. Therefore, TTFields did not induce arrhythmias and seizures.

(2) Efficacy of TTFields Compared to Conventional Chemotherapy

In 2006–2009, Stupp et al. conducted a phase III clinical trial for recurrent glioblastoma, randomly assigning 237 patients into either a TTFields treatment-only group (n = 120) or an optimal treatment group (n = 117) where the chemotherapy group was treated with the optimal regimen chosen by the physician. Results showed that the median overall survival for the TTFields group and the optimal therapy group were 16.6 months and 16.0 months, respectively

(HR = 0.86, $P = 0.27$), with 1-year survival rates of 20% and median PFS of 2.2 months and 2.1 months (HR = 0.81, $p = 0.16$), and 6-months PFS of 24.1% and 15.1% ($p = 0.16$). Quality of life assessments showed that tumor electric field therapy significantly reduced constipation, nausea, and vomiting compared to chemotherapy and helped improve cognitive function. Although the trial did not show an improvement in survival compared to conventional chemotherapy, the efficacy of the treatment was comparable, and the quality of life was significantly improved, making it a highlight of the treatment.

Mrugala et al. conducted an analysis of 457 recurrent GBM patients treated with TTFields from 91 US cancer centers via PRiDe datasets. Compared to the previous phase III trial by Stupp, a higher proportion of patients in PRiDe received TTFields for their first recurrence (33% vs. 9%) and bevacizumab treatment (55.1% vs. 19%). In clinical practice, TTFields treatment resulted in significantly longer median OS compared to the phase III trial EF-11 conducted by Stupp in 2006–2009 (9.6 months vs. 6.6 months; HR = 0.66, 95% CI: 0.05–0.86, $P = 0.0003$) and better than in patients treated with recurrent GBM in other clinical trials. The 1- and 2-year OS rates for TTFields-treated patients in PRiDe were more than twice as high as in the EF-11 trial (1-year: 44% vs. 20%). Patients with recurrent GBM and KPS $\geq$ 90 had a longer median OS (14.8 months) than those with KPS 70–80 (7.7 months), with HR = 0.6 (95% CI: 0.4–0.9, $p = 0.0070$). Higher KPS was associated with longer OS. Patients who did not receive bevacizumab had significantly longer survival compared to those who had received bevacizumab prior to starting TTFields, with median OS of 13.4 and 7.2 months, respectively. The shorter survival of patients previously treated with bevacizumab may be due to acquired tumor resistance and a more aggressive phenotype at the time of tumor progression. Patients with recurrent GBM tumors that progressed while receiving bevacizumab were often refractory to subsequent cytotoxic chemotherapy, with a median OS of only 2.7 months. It should be noted that many of the long-term survival samples mentioned in the clinical trials of bevacizumab and TMZ in recurrent GBM included small samples and were not randomized to subgroups. The results of PRiDe and those previously reported in the EF-11 trial suggest a clinical benefit of TTFields treatment in patients with recurrent GBM.

The findings indicate that TTFields treatment is well-tolerated by patients and has a favorable safety profile in clinical practice. Furthermore, no additional adverse effects were observed in PRiDe compared to the EF-11 trial. Skin reactions on the scalp beneath the electrode, which manifest as irritation and heat, remain the primary adverse effects associated with TTFields treatment. These effects can also be caused by hair, and they can be minimized by shaving the hair to re-establish optimal contact between the skin and the electrodes. Systemic adverse reactions linked to chemotherapy are rare in PRiDe datasets.

13.4 TTFields in Life Quality Assessment of GBM

The EF-14 study included health-related quality of life (HRQoL) assessments, which showed a decrease from 91.9% at baseline to 65.8% at 3 months follow-up. Patients in the TTFields-TMZ group reported an overall health status (physical condition) of 53.5% compared to 38.0% in the TMZ group ($p = 0.001$). However, overall, there were no significant differences between treatment groups in terms of HRQoL parameters, suggesting that HRQoL was similar between treatment groups for patients without tumor progression. The only significant difference was that some individuals in the TTFields group reported symptoms of scalp itching. The TTFields-TMZ group had better outcomes in terms of overall health status, physical function, emotional function, pain, and leg weakness, and the treatment did not negatively impact role and social functioning. Therefore, TTFields did not have a negative impact on quality of life at follow-up other than scalp pruritus. However, it is important to note that the lack of HRQoL data is a common limitation in many cancer clinical trials, particularly during the follow-up period, which can make the analysis of longitudinal data difficult. This limitation can result in an overrepresentation of patients with better prognostic factors and good response to treatment in later stages.

Moreover, some adjuvant medications frequently used in GBM treatment may have a negative impact on TTFields therapy. Studies have shown that immunosuppressive drugs, including dexamethasone and everolimus, may decrease the efficacy of TTFields and negatively affect patient survival. As such, it is recommended to avoid using dexamethasone or other immunosuppressive drugs in patients undergoing TTFields therapy.

13.5 Problems in TTFields Application

The delivery of TTFields therapy involves a noninvasive transducer that applies an electric field to the skin over the tumor site. The transducer is connected to a portable battery, weighing approximately 1.2 kg, which allows for continuous use of the therapy at home. In the case of GBM patients, the area of the scalp where the transducer is applied must be shaved every 3–4 days to ensure minimal surface resistance. The recommended duration of TTFields therapy is at least 18 hours per day.

Proper alignment of TTFields with the mitotic axis is critical because the non-homogeneous proximity of TTFields to cytoplasmic divisions can result in dielectric electrophoresis of charged molecules and organelles, potentially leading to mitotic disruption.

To overcome the challenge of different cell division axes in tumor tissues that can reduce the effectiveness of TTFields, a technique of sequential delivery of orthogonal and perpendicular fields by two sets of electrode pads can be used to maximize the number of tumor cells contained within the delivered TTFields. In GBM patients, individualized transducer placement is determined using MRI data to ensure maximum field strength at the target. A virtual computer model generated using finite element analysis is utilized to simulate the delivery of TTFields to the head or other anatomical regions. The TTFields settings are optimized based on the patient's unique anatomy, and the field distribution and angles generated by different locations and volumes are analyzed to achieve optimal efficacy.

Studies have demonstrated that TTFields have low systemic toxicity, and the most common adverse effect has been mild to moderate dermatitis at the site where the electrodes are placed. This is likely due to a combination of factors, including sustained moisture, heat dissipation from the skin, chemically irritating hydrogel and medical tape components, and TTFields inhibiting normal epithelial cell proliferation in the skin.

This adverse reaction was observed in 16% and 43% of patients with relapsed and newly diagnosed GBM treated with TTFields, respectively, within a timeframe of 2–6 weeks. Treatment strategies depend on the type of adverse reaction and may include topical corticosteroid creams, topical and oral antibiotics, and separation of affected skin from adhesions or compressions. Proper shaving techniques, skin care, and electrode pad displacement can prevent most of these adverse skin reactions, and effective skin care strategies can maximize patient compliance with TTFields treatment and maintain their quality of life during treatment. No serious adverse reactions associated with TTFields have been reported in any of the clinical trials conducted to date over several years of treatment. Although long-term adverse effects of TTFields may emerge in the future, current studies suggest that TTFields are well-tolerated.

There are various social and clinical factors that can influence patient adherence to TTFields therapy. While TTFields is a noninvasive treatment that allows patients to maintain their daily activities, it does require some adjustments to their lifestyle compared to traditional systemic therapy. For example, some patients may feel uncomfortable shaving their heads frequently, and wearing the electrode pads on a shaved head may make them self-conscious. Experienced healthcare providers can provide support and guidance to help patients manage these challenges and maintain their quality of life while receiving TTFields therapy. Overall, TTFields treatment is similar to oral cancer treatment in that patients can manage it at home and through outpatient care.

The adherence of patients and their caregivers is crucial for effective management of their medical condition. Several factors can influence treatment adherence, including patient-related, healthcare provider-related, and treatment-related factors. Patient-related factors such as physical limitations, psychological problems, and social issues like religion, cultural factors, and lack of systemic support can affect adherence. In contrast, healthcare providers can negatively impact adherence through poor communication, strained relationships with patients, and suboptimal treatment selection. For patients with GBM considering TTFields treatment, having a supportive family system is essential. Patients should have at least one support person who can help with equipment operation, adverse event management, scalp maintenance, and placement of electrode pads. Patients with cognitive problems or poor performance should not receive TTFields without family support. However, recent studies contradict this recommendation, showing that adherence to TTFields is independent of KPS and age and can even predict PFS and OS. Treatment-related factors such as complex treatment regimens, concomitant therapies, and adverse effects can also affect adherence. TTField treatment is unlikely to cause systemic adverse effects or affect concomitant systemic therapy.

GBM is a highly malignant tumor with a high recurrence rate and limited efficacy of conventional chemotherapy. As a result, there is an urgent need for new treatments. TTFields, a physical therapy with tumor cell specificity and tolerable adverse effects, have a solid theoretical basis and research support. In recurrent GBM, TTFields can prolong PFS and OS without adverse effects on patients. While TTFields show promising applications, some limitations need to be overcome, such as prolonged device wearing for treatment (at least 18 hours per day), a high incidence of dermatitis, and challenges in ensuring compliance. Individualized treatment protocols present a novel approach to improving clinical electric field therapy efficacy, but further research is necessary to determine their relevance to clinical antitumor efficacy.

In conclusion, TTFields represent an innovative noninvasive approach to cancer treatment. Clinical results for both primary and recurrent GBM have demonstrated its effectiveness and safety. By selectively inhibiting rapidly dividing cells through interrupting cell division, it has the potential to treat a broad range of localized tumors, including GBM. Additionally, beyond further optimization of treatment regimens for GBM, TTFields hold great promise for the treatment of other cancers.

13.6 Alternative Physiotherapy Methods

Photodynamic therapy (PDT) is an effective tumor treatment method that utilizes photosensitizer and light. The principle is that the photosensitizer accumulates specifically in glioma tumor cells through blood circulation. Under the effect of exogenous light of a specific wavelength, the photosensitizer is stimulated to produce a photodynamic reaction, leading to tumor inhibition. The photochemical reaction of PDT can directly induce tumor cell necrosis and apoptosis. Additionally, it can cause damage and occlusion of capillary endothelial cells, resulting in tumor tissue ischemia and necrosis. Furthermore, it can affect the immunogenicity of tumor cells and the progression of the tumor microenvironment, further enhancing its antitumor effect.

A phase II clinical trial of intraoperative PDT for brain tumors (including 59.1% of patients with glioblastoma) reported an overall patient survival rate of 95.5% at 12 months.

Laser interstitial thermal therapy (LITT) is a tumor treatment that uses a laser to generate high temperatures for killing tumor cells. With advancements in stereotactic and imaging technology, transcranial insertion of MRI-compatible laser catheters permits precise heat modulation through magnetic resonance temperature imaging. This enables accurate targeting and real-time monitoring of brain tumors with LITT while maximizing the protection of non-tumor brain tissue. LITT is considered a potential local treatment modality for deeply located, recurrent gliomas that are not amenable to surgery or for which standard treatment options are ineffective. It can effectively improve patient prognosis and quality of life without the risks associated with open tumor resection, shortening hospital stays and reducing hospital costs. Nevertheless, the long-term effectiveness of this treatment modality is still under evaluation through rigorous randomized clinical trials.

Focused ultrasound sonodynamic therapy, pioneered by the University of Virginia School of Medicine, employs focused ultrasound to deliver a sensitizing drug to cancer cells, which makes them susceptible to sound waves. These cells are subsequently exposed to focused ultrasound waves, creating tiny bubbles inside them that lead to cell death. This therapy shows potential as a novel treatment for gliomas. However, further clinical trials are necessary to establish its safety and efficacy.

Further Reading

Dikang C, Ling C, Yu Y. Electric field therapy for glioma. Chinese J Microinvasive Neurosurg. 2018;23(5):234–7.

Kirson ED, Dbalý V, Tovarys F, et al. Alternating electric fields arrest cell proliferation in animal tumor models and human brain tumors. Proc Natl Acad Sci U S A. 2007;104(24):10152–7.

Ma W, He H, Yu W. Advances in research on electric fields for tumor therapy. Chinese J Neurosurg. 2017;33(3):308–10.

Mrugala MM, Engelhard HH, Tran DD, et al. Corrigendum to "Clinical practice experience with novo TTFields-100A™ system for glioblastoma. The patient registry dataset (PRiDe)". Semin Oncol. 2015;42(3):e33–43.

Mun EJ, Babiker HM, Weinberg U, et al. Tumor-treating fields: a fourth modality in cancer treatment. Clin Cancer Res. 2018;24(2):266–75.

Salzberg M, Kirson E, Palti Y, et al. A pilot study with very low- intensity, intermediate-frequency electric fields in patients with locally advanced and /or metastatic solid tumors. Onkologie. 2008;31(7):362–5.

Stupp R, Wong ET, Kanner AA, et al. NovoTTF-100A versus physician's choice chemotherapy in recurrent glioblastoma: a randomised phase III trial of a novel treatment modality. Eur J Cancer. 2012;48(14):2192–202.

Stupp R, Taillibert S, Kanner AA, et al. Maintenance therapy with tumor-treating fields plus temozolomide vs temozolomide alone for glioblastoma. JAMA. 2015;314(23):2535–043.

Stupp R, Taillibert S, Kanner A, et al. Effect of tumor-treating fields plus maintenance temozolomide vs maintenance temozolomide alone on survival in patients with glioblastoma. JAMA. 2017;318(23):2306–16.

Taphoornm JB, Dirven L, Kanner AA, et al. Influence of treatment with tumor-treating fields on health-related quality of life of patients with newly diagnosed glioblastoma. JAMA Oncol. 2018;4(4):495–504.

Wong E. Tumor treating fields therapy for glioblastoma: an update. Glioma. 2019;2(2):61.

Zhu P, Zhu JJ. Tumor treating fields: a novel and effective therapy for glioblastoma: mechanism, efficacy, safety and future perspectives. Chin Clin Oncol. 2017;6(4):41.

GPSR Compliance

The European Union's (EU) General Product Safety Regulation (GPSR) is a set of rules that requires consumer products to be safe and our obligations to ensure this.

If you have any concerns about our products, you can contact us on ProductSafety@springernature.com

In case Publisher is established outside the EU, the EU authorized representative is:

Springer Nature Customer Service Center GmbH
Europaplatz 3
69115 Heidelberg, Germany

Batch number: 10731385

Printed by Printforce, the Netherlands